PRAISE FOR *THROWING THUNDER*:

"*Throwing Thunder* puts an invigorating call out to your soul to come back into sacred relationship with yourself and all of life."

RENEE BARIBEAU, AWARD-WINNING HAY HOUSE AUTHOR OF *WINDS OF SPIRIT*

"*Throwing Thunder* expresses a passionate commitment and deep concern for the authentic feminine voice, wherever it arises, whether in a person, an animal, a plant, even a weather system. This book takes a powerful stand for the transformational potency and healing necessity of that voice, celebrating the reemergence of this archetypal force in all its unpredictable wildness and beauty."

LORIE EVE DECHAR, AUTHOR OF *FIVE SPIRITS* AND *THE ALCHEMY OF INNER WORK*

"Kendra's sure feminine confidence and wildly evocative language call to a deeply soulful part of ourselves as she deftly guides us on a journey of awakening the forces of nature within. She speaks from direct experience of what it means to live with an awareness that is intimately connected to the living world and in relationship with all of life. Both practical and valuable, Kendra shows us this is a true way to be empowered as a woman."

MARY SAUNDERS, AUTHOR OF *RHYTHMS OF CHANGE*

THROWING THUNDER

Awakening the Forces of Nature Within Every Woman

Kendra Ward

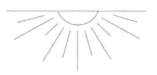

Supermoon Press
Charlotte, Vermont

Supermoon Press / Kendra Ward
P.O. Box 513
Charlotte, Vermont 05445
www.kendraward.com
permissions@kendraward.com
orders@kendraward.com

Cover design by Gus Yoo
Copy editing and book production by Stephanie Gunning

Library of Congress Control Number 2021909140

Special discounts are available to librarians and on quantity purchases by corporations, associations, and others. For details, contact the publisher at the address or website above.

Throwing Thunder / Kendra Ward —1st edition
ISBN 978-1-7370045-0-9 (paper)

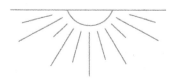

*May this writing join the growing storm of
irrepressible change roaring throughout the world,
permanently altering how women know their value
and believe themselves sacred.*

Contents

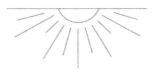

NOTE TO THE READER

Gender is infinitely complex, fluid, and deeply personal. We also know that language meant to express gender is ever changing in its cultural reflections, ultimately remaining imperfect and up for interpretation. Please know that usage of words like *woman* and *feminine* in this book are meant to be inclusive of all woman-identifying humans. At its foundation, this book is for anyone who was born from a woman, who wants to see the world through the lens of Earth-honoring, woman-respecting traditions.

INTRODUCTION

In the liminal space between waking and dreaming, I began to hear her stir. A sky creature was pacing, hungry and on the move. Hearing her slow riots of sound, I imagined that her otherworldly language could only be fully understood in the minds of earthquakes and volcanoes. The rumbling from her throat rolled and echoed through the open heavens, vibrated through my own open spaces as I lay very, very still. Reverently attentive. I waited, listening intently, for her to release her sonic shock wave of power.

I braced for her boom.

Resting in the early morning light, listening to the true nature of thunder, her behavior surprised me. Thunder does not always speak in bone-shaking, cloth-tearing, cracking, clashing cannon bursts—although she can. Her language is not always a purring, growling, shivering reverberation, leaving you expectant—although it can be. She is unpredictable, moving in her own time, at her own rhythm, a roaming changeling within a crush of cloudscapes with teachings to share—if we will listen.

Thunder makes her home in the groundless, transitory edges of space where she reminds us that we are not here to chase the passing weather of comfort or control. We are not here to be safe. We are here to risk everything and to feel exhilaratingly alive in the process.

Her presence is a shock, a wake-up call of electrical ferocity, viscerally shaking something loose in us. As her feral energy reverberates and echoes through our hollows, it excites some buried primal longing within us. Listening to her unapologetic growls connects us to the truth that we too belong to something bigger. We too crave to feel this vibrant, this free, this confident.

ix

Thunder may appear mysterious and far away from the domesticity of our everyday human lives, but she is closer than you think. She resides within the wild mesh of the natural world, a tangled, trembling, ancient system that breathes in the quiet.

We belong to this vibrating web of relationship. We are not outside its wholeness, but are intrinsically included in our awake, fascinating, pulsing, curious, living world. We are in it, of it, entrenched in its lineage even though we may have forgotten how to speak its language or respect its innate intelligence.

Nature's health is our health. Our health is nature's health. More than ever, our changing, disintegrating world is asking us to orient from this viewpoint of tender relationality. Because from somewhere not so far away, we can smell the weather changing, the winds shifting. A deep stirring, feelings of a birth coming, the labor pains of some new world moving through the pillars of our sturdy legs.

A thunderstorm is on the horizon with teachings to share. Rocking us out of assumptions and blind complacency, thunder offers us fresh perspectives on awakening our strength, autonomy, and confidence. Her power is displayed in a force of aliveness, not through power plays—power wielded over others in games of false appearances or manipulation—or worse, acts of possession, repression, terror, or scarcity. She has come to break us free—mentally, emotionally, and behaviorally—from the damaging masculine model that is our cultural norm. Thunder's voice will crumble it at its foundation.

This toxic system has convinced us that confidence is most appropriately displayed as something you assertively prop, elbow, or shove out in front of you for the effect of persuasion. There's a sense that confidence is a state of smooth certainty, completely free of doubt, that enables us to be unquestionably dominant, decisive, and self-assured. This model of confidence is so celebrated in our culture that even when you don't really feel this way, you may be encouraged to copy its guise, pumping some kind of confidence glue into the cracks of yourself to patch your imperfect exterior. We are trained to polish our masks and beautify our surfaces.

For too long, women have struggled to conform to an antiquated mold of confidence conceived by men and perpetuated through the lens of the masculine eye. Wanting to hold more power in a changing world and to feel less inhibited than we oftentimes do, women have been emulating this distorted version of confidence and critiquing ourselves harshly through its unwritten culture.

In its most extreme version, I think of expressions of female confidence as women wearing crisp power suits and assassin-sharp, bunion-generating heels. I think of complete coverage of all curves, all sway, all pop. I think of our rounded lines being forced straight, along our bodies and in our psyches. It's as if we are blotting out any undeniable mark of our femininity on the page of ourselves with dirty erasers, leaving some smudged confusion—and a twisting in our guts.

Like circles being stuffed into square holes, women for decades have attempted to disguise our differences in order to gain belonging as a plastic army of pseudo-men, morphed into something strange and unnatural. Despite gradual, nominal changes to this hulking system, the slippery, lingering imprints of cultural expectation drift in us somewhere still, unconsciously internalized.

Listing in an ocean of possibility polluted by the floating trash of the patriarchy, we are slowly strangled by an old ideology too slow to break down. Our lack of progress in gaining genuine parity with men over the last century owes much to some stubborn refusal of these beliefs to decompose.

Some of us are stirring, nonetheless. There is a growing awakening among women that past paradigms centered around confidence are tired and obsolete. But what does the true embodiment of confidence look and feel like for the modern woman? At some point, this question began moving in me—thunder's storm of inquiry, charged and restless in my mind. I began to listen for the voice of confidence all around me, asking confidence what she wanted to teach me, what new viewpoint she wanted to emerge.

Asking again and again: What would it look like to be lit up with it—to radiate confidence from the inside out?

Thunder guided me to turn this question over to the collective and that's why I present here to you. In this moment, on this planet home, what is our best female avatar of healthy, spirit-fueled, root-based confidence? Not in a masked, looking-good-on-the-outside, but shivering-with-self-loathing-on-the-inside kind of way.

Not in a threateningly insecure or wear-too-much-red kind of way either.

Not in a "learn to flirt better" or "get a promotion at work" way.

Not in any skin-deep, ego-propping-up ways—not even as badass boss babes ruling the room or making multimillion-dollar business deals before breakfast.

As sexy and enticing as these examples may appear to us, they reflect how easily we are lured back into a masculine paradigm of forcing, proving, or dominating our way through the world. They promote a sense of being untouchable, unstoppable, impenetrable.

But do we really want to be that hardened?

I have concluded that a feminine paradigm of confidence thrives in acts of vulnerability, authenticity, and trust, a softening of our heavy armor and all of the ways we thought we had to fight our way through our lives. And I am interested in a confidence that is more persistent and long-lasting, whose resilience lingers beyond sweet surges of feeling invincible or days you feel crushed on the rocks of hopelessness.

What exists beyond the roller-coaster ride of unreliable old-fashioned confidence? The ups and downs of a confidence that is only surface scratching—and not soul-seeded—make us feel sick and unrooted. This old model just cannot endure.

Superficial confidence has us always asking: When will it be enough? In all of our strivings, pushings, provings, and other doings we are constantly seeking to find our worth outside of ourselves. Smacking up against wall after wall of self-doubt, pooling in puddles of exhaustion, we have to be willing to finally look within.

The rebellious sounds of thunder pound again, reminding us that we can change the way we have been relating to confidence. We can invent something new. We no longer need to understand and evaluate our confidence through a masculine model that just doesn't fit. In the pages of this book, it is my intention to challenge you to rethink your motivations. Instead of always trying to change ourselves, persuaded into more unhealthy shapeshifting, let us reimagine our relationship with confidence as something that more fiercely claims our full expression as women.

Thunder's Wake-Up Call

Thunder's voice is endlessly creative and varied, but her signature display of raw power comes in hooves, a tremendous migration of stampeding buffalos across the sky. This is a sound that makes your eyes widen and pulse quicken; it grabs you and jolts you out of complacency and numbness. It is not a sound you can sleep through.

It is a shock wave of awakening. Thunder as the fierce revolutionary, wants us to change the rules and think outside the bounds of our everyday perceptions. Her call to action challenges our assumptions, all of the ways we have been living while asleep. Beyond having too much or too little confidence, thunder wants us to better understand our *unexamined* confidence. For the constant static of distraction in our busy lives keeps us easily focused elsewhere. This lack of honest inquiry leaves our confidence imprisoned as a frail and fickle creature of sorts. It can feel safer sometimes for us to ignore it altogether, a quiet, assumed hope in its sturdy existence.

But in this call of aliveness, thunder reminds us that healthy confidence belongs to all of us. It is not a shallow indulgence, but a *profound spiritual need*. Our confidence—or lack of it—impacts everything in our lives, shaping how we speak, how we interact, and what we think is possible for ourselves. It is contagious and inspiring, putting its persuasive, powerful imprint on everything in our lives.

As part of making confidence our own, we come to see that it is not something we can lasso down through more mental sweat and rumination. It is not something outside of us that we need to buy, copy, fake, or wrestle with. It lives in us. Waiting patiently. Wanting us to awaken, touch, feel, feed, listen to, and trust its essence. We must be willing to hear its thunderous voice and feel its urgings within us. We have to be ready to finally recognize that it is there, wanting to interact with us fully.

My Thunder

I come to these confidence inquiries as a fellow traveler but also as a witness and teacher. After having spent close to the last two decades working as an acupuncturist and herbalist, I have held space for thousands and thousands of women to express and explore the deepest part of their lives: their bodies' wise teachings, their heartaches, their celebrations, the deaths and births of their children and their creative projects, as well as the things they may never tell other people. During these years, I have been equally humbled by the tremendous depth of women's suffering and the brightness of their ceaseless inner light.

It is because of these women that I moved into action. Some fire was lit in me along with a realization that I had never really felt like confidence belonged to me fully. It always remained slightly elusive, just out of reach.

I have heard this same description from so many other women. Reflecting on its true nature, I have come to believe that wounds to our core confidence are actually *the beating heart* of our struggles as women today. They're getting in the way of our ability to contribute what we have to the world. They hold us back, individually and collectively.

And this has got to finally shift.

That's the ultimate purpose of what is gathered here: to initiate and propel change.

Core confidence wounds have a way of showing up at every twist and turn. Perhaps for you personally this emerges during an attempt to leave a stale, unfulfilling job, or in the shadows of your most intimate relationships, or in your desire and ability to initiate creative endeavors—in any kind of edge-walking you do, period.

We need to address—and mend—the gaping confidence wounds that too many women incur as a result of not feeling genuinely worthy as human beings. Imagine how much beauty, brilliance, and wisdom this world would gain if we shared our loves and talents more openly?

It is shocking to contemplate how, throughout the history of civilization, up to the present day, we have been missing out on experiencing the full advantages of feminine contribution. Think of all the art, science, literature, spiritual guidance, and more that was never born because women's voices were silenced, their bodies constrained and controlled. All those thousands of years of potential insight now gone, because women were told it was not their place.

We have gotten so numbed out to this truth that we may have never let the immensity of our loss sink in.

The world faces tremendous challenges today because of this missing female intelligence, in politics and decision-making, in industry and innovation, even in fields that we stereotypically think of as being more archetypally or conventionally feminine, a deficiency *still* looms. It is a weeping wound, purulent yet active, ever working through various stages of hope and mending.

All subversive change comes with a shift in seeing, a deeper listening.

Have you really listened to thunder, or to what is wild in you?

The movement of thunder is an unapologetic, untamed, and free-spirited force. Let us pull the energy of thunder deep within us, letting it become our own, shaking all of the things in our lives loose that keep us feeling small and powerless. Learning the language of thunder, let it speak a different version of confidence to us, a "feminine confidence" that wants room to stretch, to breath, to move freely within us. Out of its dark waters there arises a sense of unlimited potential, the seeds for life, the laws of nature, the creation of cycles, and a knowing of our own rhythms.

Feminine confidence has space for all of us, even our fears and doubts. It encourages us to stop questioning ourselves all of the time and to take up the habit of honoring our gut impulses. Unafraid of our desires, our thirsts, our tender vulnerabilities, this is an instinctual, Earth-based confidence that awakens and liberates the forces of nature every woman already carries within her.

What Swells Within You

These may be uncharted territories, but we don't need to go it alone. We will use the guidance and support of four particular archetypes as a way to better understand the many varied expressions of feminine confidence. After learning to connect with these energies within ourselves, we will call on them throughout the rest of our confidence inquiries and use them in practices and journaling questions.

Following the spiral path of our human experience, we will trace feminine confidence through the body, mind, heart, soul, and all of the connecting points between them. Beginning with the realm of our flesh, we will find that healthy embodiment acts as one of the many keys of genuine confidence, offering us opportunities to look deeper into behaviors of shame, unconscious body-apologizing and shield wearing. The sound of these writings is a thunder that wakes you up, electrifies the hairs along your skin, reminding you that you have this gift of a body, that you are alive.

In the realm of the mind, we find that confidence does not always come to us through life feeling comfortable or familiar; sometimes we must come to know feminine confidence through periods of sacred initiation, feeling broken, lost, and discovering an unshakeable resilience. This is a confidence that is built on a vigorous engagement with difficulty—a teaching of how oftentimes we learn more in the darkness of our lives than in the light. The sound of these writings is a thunder that comes hard and heavy with unrelenting acoustics that ricochet and rumble through our skulls, but then unexpectedly dies into a quivering peace.

In the realm of the heart, we are reminded of the interpersonal, interglobal, intergalactic power of love and the ways that we may still believe it does not belong to us fully. When we approach self-compassion more carefully, we come to find that it is not this squishy, naïve thing unfit to stand up to the real world, but that it is fierce and durable, a kind of forceful self-loyalty we can return to again and again. Feeding ourselves on love and compassion fills our deep inner wells with a richness and sufficiency. The sound of these writings is a thunder like a drumbeat, steady low rumbles continually rippling through your chest and heart.

In the realm of the soul, we find the confidence to look at how busyness acts as a clever distraction from accessing the deeper layers of ourselves. We come to honestly see how we hide behind our doings and our givings as proof of our self-worth. The confidence of a soul-led woman knows how to rest, receive, lay down and trust in her life. The sound of these writings is a thunder that cracks and then waits, interspersed by long periods of drenching, rejuvenating rain.

The dark feminine path asks for unrelenting authenticity and radical self-responsibility. I offer you no smug assumptions or plastic-wrapped definitions of confidence to be uncovered in snappy three-step plans or dumbed-down listicles. I will not pretend that I can hand confidence to you in a perfectly wrapped box with polka-dot paper and a smooth satin ribbon. Disrupting the ways that you have thought about confidence in the past, I want you to find its current truths for yourself. Introspective questioning and journaling opportunities shift these writings from remaining conceptual philosophies alone, moving you into the legitimacy of your own trial and error, your own lived and embodied experience.

Along the way you may discover that ongoing experimentation is more interesting than pretending like you have everything figured out. Layered with rich, contemplative substance, these writings seek to convince you that knotty enigmas and playful paradox are more intriguing than certainty. Let these questionings have life, let them have teeth, biting into the heart of the matter, juices of inspiration and honesty running down our faces, sticky and persistent.

Woman, you are a vast storm of possibility. Do not be scared of what swells within you. I see your clouds forming like large pieces of sliced agate in the sky, bands of gray, pale purple, and gold. I sense all that you possess: a rumbling of electricity and excitement, mystery and sovereignty. I also feel the ways in which you have been reigned in until now, the barometric pressure of your self-doubt and fear. There is wisdom in this wild tempest, a slow swirling growing with all you hold: wrathful feminine, seductive feminine, ambivalent feminine, infinite feminine.

The crash and boom of thunder are meant to wake us out of our complacency. This gathering energy holds the promise of release, the hope of revitalization, and the exhilarating freshness of freedom. But you cannot skip the storm. No, you cannot have the rainbow without that transformative rain.

When will you let us feel all you've got? Instead of battening the hatches down tighter or hiding out in your bunker, it is time to pound us with your hail, baptize us anew with your purifying downpour, to finally throw down your thunder. Because waiting in the calm eye of this storm is the light of your natural confidence, the truth of all you contain.

CHAPTER ONE

Feminine Confidence

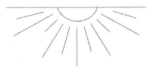

"The old one, The One who Knows, is within us. She thrives in the deepest soul-psyche of women, the ancient and vital wild Self. Her home is that place in time where the spirit of women and the spirit of wolf meet—the place where mind and instincts mingle, where a woman's deep life funds her mundane life." [1]
—CLARISSA PINKOLA ESTÉS

There is a naturally arising confidence that comes from believing in our wholeness. This is the same wholeness that we share with a purple aster, born to turn its resplendent face up towards the sky. It is the same wholeness of lavender mist sunrises and fiery amber sunsets, perfect drops of rainwater on lupine leaves, and a billion other acts of rebellious beauty. This earth-based model of confidence includes you in its understanding of inherent completeness, despite your fears, your doubts, your imperfections, or your insecurities. Despite all of the ways you might try to keep yourself separate and outside of its naturalness.

Confidence Reimagined

Awakening from our previous conditioning and default assumptions, let us first aim to understand the essence of feminine confidence so that we can better recognize it and claim it within ourselves. Shifting our allegiances away from an antiquated system of confidence that perpetuates some façade of polished appearances, while barely covering parched and shaky cores, feminine confidence graciously welcomes all aspects of ourselves. Refusing to participate in these old narratives of persuasion opens space to reimagine a feminine confidence fed by subversively returning to ourselves with compassion and loyalty, over and over again.

Feminine confidence is characterized by a woman who is patiently gathering her tempest. A deluge may be coming.

Or she is a woman who has drawn in the breath of her squall, allowing herself to feel an absence of urgency, a refusal to distractedly rush or push.

She may feel honey-sweet and well-behaved in one moment and then flash her jagged, thunder bolt teeth at you in the next.

She can be easy sunshine, a thrashing monsoon, well-behaved breezes, furious hail, and everything in between. Feminine confidence accommodates your full range of weather patterns—and finds them exciting and creative.

Now, the term *feminine confidence* works beautifully for holding the essence of what I am trying to express, although I would admit that it still holds the potential for endless misinterpretation. Honestly, even the word *confidence* is super loaded and uncomfortable for many women, who may sense it as some form of thoughtless bravado. Seen in its most ugly, aggressive forms, forced confidence can make us squirm with its false, disingenuous front.

The Latin root of the word *confidence, confidentia,* means "firmly trusting or to have full reliance."[2] Confidence is about boldly believing in something. Feeling its truth settle, *kerplunk,* deep into the center of you, let this be a fierce belief in yourself. And realizing that genuine confidence is not built on pomp and noise but on the much more eternal column of your own radical self-trust.

Radical implies an audacity, a rawness, a revolt against what we assume robotically or habitually. It is naive to assume that the honesty of feminine confidence is easy to constantly embody. It is not so simple to live at the crux of your authenticity, knowing with conviction the truth that lies at the sacred intersection of your humanity and your divinity.

It requires genuine acts of courage from us.

But *confidence* isn't the only word that comes with a backpack of baggage. I would also like to liberate the word *feminine,* especially from our standard associations of it with adjectives like *tender, ladylike,* and *soft,* which hold the assumption of softness as a form of weakness, lying in direct opposition of confidence. I am not interested in these stark polarities, the ways in which we keep trying to deny that both masculine and feminine forces live in all of us.

Instead, the word *feminine* in the phrase *feminine confidence* speaks to a power that comes from the vast cosmic ocean of being and creation. It is out of these black seas that there arises a sense of deep time, unlimited potential, the endless genius of nature, and the constant, dynamic flux of change. This great incubator holds the embryonic seeds for the infinite diversity of life out of which we co-arise.

All beings come from and are a part of this mysterious feminine, this fertile vat of complete totality. It is a force so much bigger than our tendency to want to pit men against women, women against men.

Which prompts me to wonder where the true intersection of femininity and confidence is located? Imagine a concept embracing dualities that push and play off of each other like rascals: gentle and bold, trusting and courageous, wild and disciplined, free and committed. These are the junctions of possibility I like to explore, the places where we can begin to understand what it means to be a woman wielding her inner thunder well. These are the evolutionary tides, the fertile creative grounds where, out of the void, a new story can be birthed.

Discovering the nature of feminine confidence for yourself is about standing in the dark of your storm and doing some deep listening. This is a different kind of listening, a tuning in beyond words that follows the arc of emotion leading directly to the soul. It is driven by a hunger to better understand what dwells beneath the surface of things, digging deeper to become increasingly clear on how and why you disempower yourself, if and when you do. It is about taking ownership of your Earth walk while it lasts.

I contend there is a naturally intelligent confidence that already lives within you. Just like your own feminine nature, it is deeply personal and hard to define. This confidence knows that unworthiness does not exist in the natural world and that your birthright is this model. It wants room to breathe and roam freely. No added glitz needed to know it or turn it on. But you do need to acknowledge its presence. It wants to be felt and known.

Moving forward, I will be using the term *feminine confidence* as a definition that best expresses this newly invented version of confidence—one that makes better room for our full experience as women.

How to Feed a Woman

Feminine confidence wants us to know what really feeds us as women. It wants us to find depth in our understanding of the true nature of nourishment and self-care. More sturdy and unwavering than old structures of confidence, feminine confidence connects us to our primal longings and essential desires. It wants us to indulge our voracious appetites for life.

It can be hard to interpret what really feeds us with the women's health industry constantly shouting all sorts of consumerism-based self-care ideas to women through magazine headlines, TV commercials, and billboards.

We are fed the dirty lie that "self-care" is found in spa days, the latest facials, chocolate bars, perfumes, lotions, mattresses, mani-pedis, hair coloring, bath salts, fancy shoes—in shopping "therapy." An entire industry markets itself on catching the rebellious heart strings of women, telling them that they are "worth it" —worth the indulgence, the purchase, the splurge.

We are manipulated into believing that we can buy our way into deep soul sustenance. But all of this surface-scratching consumerism leaves us empty and still searching. How do we really feed a woman?

How do we sustain ourselves in a way that is soul deep, with a sweet nectar lovingly poured into our inner well? What is this spirit food based in and where does it come from?

These questions seem to be able to stop even the most accomplished, intelligent, well-put-together woman in her tracks. For there are thousands of ways to seek mediocre nourishment, but it is more challenging to connect with the things that genuinely enrich our lives. The truth is that most of us skim the surface of sustenance from our choices in life: the people, the food, the images, the entertainment, and the environments we choose to engage in.

Authentic nutrition comes from feeding the animal spirit of a woman. Her curious heart needs more than the skin deep, needs more than just temporary pleasure. She is tired of her training in restriction and domestication, becoming increasingly numb to the stirrings and the rumblings within. These are the yearnings that she may be too afraid to feel, the ways in which she may not even recognize herself anymore.

In the past it may have been far easier for her to just fit herself into the system as it was, despite its soul-crushing repercussions. The constraints and expectations of our familial or cultural systems, the pace, the distractions, the orientation of our modern lives have all taught us to withhold.

Taught us to take too little or nothing at all.

Taught us to receive too little dreaming, too little creativity, too little spaciousness, too little love, too little breath, too little passion, too little trust, too little freedom.

When we allow ourselves to be open to feeling and hearing this animal spirit within, we realize that we crave a tremendous stretch of our spirits. We begin to remember that life is supposed to feel good to us. Not in some perfect, hedonistic, always go our way kind-of-good. But that our default mode does not need to be some withholding of goodness, joy, delight, and beauty. That we can receive more fully.

Our Instinctual Nature

True freedom as women relies on being in touch with our instinctual nature and knowing how to care for the longings of our souls. What a tremendous relief to be able to let the soul lead, to have ears that recognize its howl and chirp, fingers that know its fur and feathers. A soul-led life asks us to bypass the over intellectualization of our experience and to let some gut-level, primordial power come forward. It asks us to leave our early training and reliance on abstract reasoning and to let something more ancient and intuitive guide us.

There is this instinctual woman in you, always there, always longing for contact.

She is always waiting for you. Under your junk emails and sticky dishes piled in the sink, she is waiting. Under the schedule that wants to sprint away from you, beneath your maze of distractions and impatient errand running, she is waiting.

There is a soft whispering in your ear as she speaks softly, but persistently to you. She reminds you that there are clouds galloping past the daytime moon, improvisational dancers of light decorating your walls, and entire universes living below your feet. Feel her there on the fringes, in whispers and the wind, on the edge of your shoulder, just grazing your consciousness. She is easiest to find in the liminal spaces, the borderlands between waking and dreaming, the margins of night and day, in the shadowy haze and eerie hush of the gloaming.

The instinctual woman also dwells in the sudden, shocking transitions of life, those moments that untether you from your everyday reality, the stake poles of your life lifted, turning what you thought was solid into infinite floating specks. You may feel her presence stronger in times of great beauty and peak experience, as well as in moments of raw pain, when she collects the bones of your suffering. She lives in the breathing quiet of the transitory places where you intersect with your essence.

You might look for her—

In the empty space between the dark matter mesh of the cosmos.

Through the alert eyes of an osprey high atop a grandfather redwood.

In the moan and stretch of glacial ice, alive and creeping.

From the back of a blue whale sounding, diving deeper into the black.

In the warm breath of the wolf as she breaks trail through fresh, playful snow.

The resonance of these places lives out there and also in us.

But invoking the wisdom of the instinctual woman does not need to feel exotic or based in a distant wilderness. Connecting with her spirit brings us back to the memory that woven into the very core of our being are all of the elements of nature. The wisdom of the Earth is deeply embedded into our cells and it is here that our tattered nervous systems can be truly cradled in a hammock of belonging. It is here that we can let our heart-roots, the roots of our truths, grow thick and sturdy, plunging into the black, mother dirt.

Animal Longings

Instead of quietly suffering alone, persuaded to starve our wildness, we are asked to rearrange our priorities. This wise and warrior-like part of ourselves reminds us to protect our time and energy—to fend off the things that threaten our joy, rapture, and astonishment with sharp claws.

The instinctual woman within us begins to rebel when we are cut off from our creative source, when we care too much, try too hard, are too nice. All of these tenuous provings of our worth keep our confidence flimsy, untrustworthy, and contingent on the opinions of others.

Often she is speaking within us, but we have trained ourselves to ignore her voice or tune out the grumblings of her hunger pains. I feel her unacknowledged appetite in myself at times and in many of the women I know.

I notice the stirrings of primal longing in a woman who is a slave to her job, aware deep-down of how stuck and muzzled she feels, who remains too afraid to challenge the comforts of her familiar lifestyle.

I watch the instinctual animal within whine to be released in a woman who must clean her house from top to bottom before she can allow herself to play in her painting studio.

I see wings want to sprout from the back of a woman moving through a mid-life transition, suddenly throwing herself up against the bars of her self-imposed prison, cursing how everyone and everything else's needs always come before her own.

When you make contact with the instinctual woman within and allow yourself to be fully released and utterly alive, you become allergic to a too-small-existence and the starvation of your spirit. You may come to feel that you cannot bear to live a life that doesn't honor this freedom. In the past you may have spent time stuck in the wastelands of shallow strivings, but you now know that you never want to return to those soul deserts again.

When you deeply know where this grounded, raw, animalistic confidence lives in you, it is less scary to touch into those parts of yourself that are feral, maybe even a little dark, a little dangerous. As part of your inheritance within the continuum of the living world, you listen to the language of nature and come to know how to put out your own strange call. Your animal ears perk up hearing and waiting for the song of every creature in return.

You feel the vibration held within the plants and animals and know how to shiver and speak back to them. It is in this mutual recognition that human words no longer want to come, in an intelligence that is so much less primitive than the rational modern present. As a woman who relies on her instincts, you understand the tongue of thunder and lightning, the dialect of watchful stars, and the commands of almighty earthquakes. You remember that in every culture around the world, the voice of the feminine emerges from the land itself.

When you are very quiet, you can feel how you belong to something so much bigger. Your soul asks you to perceive a multidimensional viewpoint, knowing that you are so much more than this brief, physical body. You are an archeologist of mystery, carrying the dust of something primordial and indestructible in your core. You hear the drumbeats of your Earth-honoring ancestors, those that lived well and died well, and draw their wisdom and guidance into your heart.

The instinctual woman is there with you when you are walking the steepest mountain edges, wandering through forgotten forests, when you feel so completely lost, so completely broken that you finally perceive the deeper strength and sustenance of your resilience. She is there in the ravages of grief when you tear at your hair or hang heavy as a heap of rags on the floor. She is with you in all your various phases of painful becoming.

The instinctual woman in you is fed on daily connections to her essential longings, the desires that unite you with your core values and driving force.

She nourishes you in a sense of belonging, to other humans, to the land where you live, to the vast living world. You are a root among many millions of roots growing in one breathing, pulsing, entangled web.

She moves you towards freedom, galloping your sleek mustang over the golden hills of wonder and awe. There may have been a life that you numbly, unconsciously chose years ago, but you know you no longer need to keep yourself small for its sake.

She sustains you by knowing yourself as possible. You feel possible to yourself when you have the confidence to do something differently than you might have done in the past. When you are the architect of your destiny, you remember that conscious choice is the greatest power you possess.

Look for her now. Listen for her. Slow down for her. She lives in you; she has all along. She will never stop wanting to connect. Her loving whispers will never cease.

The Spiral Dance

The instinctual woman is the soul-source of our feminine confidence. She trusts in the movement of life. Self-inquiry reminds us of both her dark and bright aspects, flesh and spirit, and her evolution through the symbolic spiral of self-discovery. Journeying through the cycles of the spiral is to resonate with the pleasure of living, stages of aging, faith in being, and trust in life as it is.

It is through the spiral that we remember to submerge ourselves in the currents of the animate world. Instead of always watching our life go by as if stuck behind the safety and sterility of a windowpane, we must open the window of ourselves and let the cathartic, tempestuous winds blow through. This call to aliveness wants to flash through our senses, flow over our skin, expand our pores, dilate our pupils, and thrash our hair about. Moving this current into our bodies, we feel its vitality course through our electric channels. Our inner ecology wants us to stand in this flux of aliveness and let it rush through and all around us.

It is in the spiral that the instinctual woman sees the legitimacy of all beings around her. She watches the urge in all things to move towards life, the push of aliveness in a growing seedling, a growing child, growing dreams, even a growing universe. She trusts in life, trusts in change, trusts in love, trusts in knowing when to hold tight and when to let go.

Connecting with the symbol of the spiral has awakened some inherent mystery within people throughout the ages of human history. We can find evidence of the spiral in ancient and indigenous art ranging from the carvings of Bronze Age stones at Newgrange in Ireland to the paintings of Australian Aborigines.

When we see nature dance and rejoice in this universal design element, it is awe inspiring. The sacred geometry of spirals are everywhere: in the shell of a snail, the head of a Romanesco cauliflower, the unfolding of a rose, the tail of a chameleon, a freshly curled fiddlehead fern, a cyclonic storm on Jupiter, a threatening coastal hurricane, the face of a sunflower, bathwater spinning down a drain, and the Pinwheel Galaxy.[3] It is a symbol that links the microcosm, like the whorls on our fingerprints, to the macrocosm of the largest swirling galaxies.

The spiral encourages us to hold our noses and jump with both feet into the cauldron of darkness: the feminine black of possibility.

Here the great mystery teaches us a reverence for the painful beauty in all of the mundane miracles of everyday life. Here we find a beauty that hurts. These are the moments that openly tenderize us with the gorgeousness of life, keep us wishing we could hold on to them, just as they are, forever. But this beauty is meant to be fleeting. It is meant to pierce us and keep our blood moving.

We find painful beauty in the apprehension of an autumn gingko about to drop her blazing yellow gown of leaves, poised for sudden nakedness. We watch it in the trembling white skin of the moon as she falls into the loyal arms of the sea. We feel its transience in early morning mountain silhouettes, supernatural pastels of blush pink and rose gold that quickly transform into the colors of full daylight. It is a beauty that squeezes our lungs, brings tears to our eyes, grips our tender insides. This beauty thunders and races across the plains of our hearts, feral and uncatchable.

Dancing the path of the spiral, we find ourselves part of this impermanent, quivering lattice of life. We do not forget the soft ache of our brief existence. We know our lives as sacred. Looking up and around, we appreciate and take pleasure in the absurd possibility that we live on a Goldilocks planet—a ball of rock hurtling through space that's just the right distance from a sun to grow life but not fry all of that life to a crisp. The spiral reminds us that we are part of this miracle and so many more, that the flow of the great mystery powerfully moves within us and all around us.

Because really there are no straight lines in the living world. Even the lines that we perceive on a tree or a leaf always have a slight bend to them. Even what seems to be the most inescapable lines in nature, like the horizon, are not lines at all, but a gentle curve of a certain diameter that is impossible to perceive with the naked eye. It is us humans that have designed lives made with straight and tidy rows, always ready to box up what wants to run free.

The living world stretches, slithers, flows, and rotates. With each turn of the spiral, we discover what circles and moves in us and we better understand that to which we return. We more clearly discern our daily choices and what we come home to, in our habits, in our behaviors, in our thoughts. Every day our instinctive nature wants us to move towards what makes us feel viscerally alive and whole.

Are we returning to—

Opening or shutting down?

Self-criticism or self-loyalty?

Inner-persecution or grace?

What is worthy of us circling back to? This rhythmic spiraling towards feminine confidence allows for authentic transformation and sustained change, moving us ever closer to a truer version of ourselves.

A Glorious Force

Traveling through the unfurling spiral, we are reminded how healthy confidence touches everything in our lives: Its love mists our faces. Its bounty fills the cups of those closest to us. Its richness nourishes our creative impulses. Its moisture quenches our connections and work, encouraging sanity and health.

Remember, in a way, feminine confidence functions like echo-location. Similar to the sound waves that are given off by dolphins, bats, and certain kinds of birds, the confidence we emit bounces back to us, helping us orient ourselves. This vibration speaks of our openness, our curiosity, and the willingness of our hearts to expand their apertures rather than doing another hard contraction. And when we approach our relationships with a sense of availability, others sense it. Feminine confidence allows us to interact with integrity, orienting our relationships from a place of inspiration that opens us to receive the best from others.

When you inspire someone, they feel excited by your energy, presence, and special genius. Your energy uplifts them, helping them feel encouraged, creative, or positively provoked into action. And they do the same for you.

Feminine confidence isn't about walking into a room and thinking you are better than everyone else; it's walking into a room and not needing to compare yourself to anyone at all. When you feel truly steady within yourself, you don't need anyone to prop you up or anyone to stand on top of. You can stand your ground as a sovereign being.

The world desperately needs us to express our unapologetic autonomy. It wants more of us. Not in a greedy, life-sucking sort of way but in a flourishing, generous, full-belly way. It wants us to boldly take up space. The greater mystery is in cahoots with us, rooting for us, wanting all of us. Without doing our work to develop a strong sense of feminine confidence rooted in feelings of self-worth, we will always feel socially and spiritually vulnerable, and a feeling of perpetual lack will persist. But a confident woman who knows her value, despite everything life throws at her, is a glorious and furious force like no other.

CHAPTER TWO

Storm of Inquiry

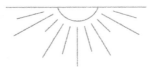

"Once upon a time, when women were birds, there was the simple understanding that to sing at dawn and to sing at dusk was to heal the world through joy. The birds still remember what we have forgotten, that the world is meant to be celebrated."[1]

—TERRY TEMPEST WILLIAMS

Mottled brown feathers so ingeniously camouflaged, body so still and reverent, it would have completely evaded detection if it hadn't been for my son's bright eyes.

Inherent Trust

One half avian wizardry, one half smoky enigma, the well-disguised ghost of a bird immediately fixed its radar dish upon us. In turn, it was impossible for us to pull away from the fluid, supernatural movements of this large owl, its eyes like black saucers of deep space.

We stopped moving and hovered to observe it, minds entranced and voices hushed.

Just being in the bird's presence was a chance to touch the depths of a quality of nature that we so infrequently experience, a wildness without names, labels, or words. The owl's silence seemed to speak of something feral and fierce, overgrown and uninhabited, and also continuously, flowing and living within us too.

There was the stirring of dark kinship.

The shadowy striations along the owl's plumage seemed to swell and surge like muscles flexed as its feathers fluffed and then settled back down again.

Rouse. Rest.

A kindly breeze came running its currents through each barred layer, exciting feathers that had just laid down, resolved.

Rouse. Rest.

Time lazed and lengthened, almost on the verge of a nap, only to be shocked precise again by a quick snap of the bird's head reacting to some stealth movement below.

Rouse. Rest.

Then there was some in-between state, neither rousing nor resting, but an active attention blended with a sense of effortlessness accompanying the relaxed mastery of simply sitting on a branch.

Maintaining a loose watchfulness and open availability to the teaching of the bird's tremendous natural power, I observed how its every plume communicated an inherent authority and ease within itself. Which sounds funny to say (because it's an owl, for Pete's sake), but the truth is that we do not get many examples of this kind of simple self-assurance in the human realm.

This kind of honest confidence seems to shine so easily from the bodies of animals. A lioness is not thinking her way through her easy swagger, through her resounding growl—they are just in her. And a dolphin is not thinking her way through her skill with the waves—it just moves through and out of her.

Animals express the kind of confidence that is innate. Unforced and even unassuming, this confidence presses itself on no one. It just is.

We know it when we see it.

Even in humans, we know it in essence, in voice, in posture. We feel it in the tones and textures of energy, in the walk and poise of body language, and maybe even in the vague lingering of certain smells.

But simple self-assurance gets much more complicated with us big-brained mammals. Confidence goes from being intrinsic and unquestioned to something a lot more murky and slippery to grasp. At times we may think we have gotten hold of some version of it, only to have it become slick and sliding out of reach once more.

What is crystal clear is that each of us entered this world confident and at ease within ourselves. There is nothing shifty or uncertain about the granite boulder-like confidence firmly lodged into the core of us at our birth. Chiseled in bold script somewhere on this mighty rock, I imagine the words *I am complete. I am love.*

But somehow over time the weathering and wear of life erodes this stone of absoluteness, mostly with other mind carvings—often some version of *I am not enough.* What appears so plain, so incontestable, so smack-you-in-the-face obvious at the beginning of our lives—this integral confidence—gets slowly reworked and reinscribed over time.

Wholeness still exists in us somewhere, closer than we think. It is not outside of us but imbued in our fibers and viscera, unable to ever be dissected or peeled away. Just like any other animal, we belong to nature. We belong to this wholeness. The living world reminds us to bask in our uncomplicated completeness. But because we position ourselves outside of nature, we are unable to see ourselves as a continuance of all living things. We are disconnected from understanding how her primal powers govern our inner ecology. Without realizing it, we may think of ourselves as observers, manipulators, worshippers, purchasers of nature, failing to see ourselves within her still—and therefore seeing ourselves as less than whole.

Robotically operating with an attitude of ownership instead of respectful relationship, we continually try to separate and elevate ourselves above the womb of all being. Somehow, we have come to believe in the deceptive mirage that one creature can reign supreme from all of the vastly woven living world—a world that it is intricately a part of and on which it relies for its very life.

Something about this particular bird encounter lingered with me. Resting there in the bright sunlight of midday, its branch hanging over a busy hiking trail, it did not fly away. It just stayed and stayed. As people wandered by, unimpressed, its presence began to feel just for me. This bird teacher was showing me what it means to be completely relaxed within oneself—a natural confidence based in inherent trust.

Enamored by the owl's presence, this was the beginning of a shift in my awareness and the start of my longing to better understand where authentic confidence lies. Transforming our viewpoint and knowing ourselves as knitted within the vibrant web of nature, we are reminded that confidence is potentially our truest, most genuine state of being.

What Does Your Confidence Rest On?

Dog hair tumbleweeds and daddy long leg webs gather in stopping points, the quiet paralysis of the corners of my home. On my hands and knees, I wipe, I vacuum, I scrub, reaching the familiar places I've washed clean before. But there is always that stopping point, that border in the dust, those places just beyond the reach of my arm. Under the bed, the couch, the fridge, I am suddenly aware of all that remains untouched in the spaces I thought were so clean.

Our inner selves are similarly dusty. We all have places and beliefs within us that remain unexamined, sometimes in blindingly clear sight, just out of reach. These stories and thought patterns stubbornly persist because it is too hard, too familiar, too painful, or too uncomfortable to investigate them. We might see our dark storm of inner inquiry, brewing and waiting across the horizon but we may feel too intimidated to approach it, too scared to proceed.

Kind and skillful questioning unlocks learning within us, asking us to uncover what we might have known all along. This is our intent: to finally perceive what lingers in the dim corners of our minds and intuition, knowing that stormy weather draws something different from us than clear blue skies. There is some needed cleanse within the center of those thunderheads. So, I ask you now:

What has drawn you to these confidence inquiries?

How do you view your confidence in your life right now?

There will be further opportunities to creatively explore these questions in greater depth at the end of the chapter but for now, grow this open curiosity in yourself.

There is no one set way that we struggle with confidence, but these are a few common situations that I observe frequently:

- Women who recognize the importance of confidence but feel intimidated by it, to the point that it feels distant and unreachable. Entirely unrelatable and unreliable. Hands might get thrown up in the air with a *why bother* shrug.
- Women whose confidence is entirely situational, based on some other person or external circumstance. They may feel fine, sturdy even, when it comes to doing something they've practiced a zillion times, but they quickly whip into a tornado of self-deprecation as soon as they feel out of their element in any way.
- Women who feel turned off by the idea of confidence in general and all that it might represent. This is the struggle to see or feel confidence outside of the past associations we have, and perhaps

for good reason. A modern thesaurus still gives us words like *cocksure* and *presumptuous* when we search for synonyms for *confident*.[2] Who wouldn't want to turn around and run away screaming from associating themselves with that version of confidence?

- Women who haven't had reason to give their confidence much thought recently. Or even if they have a vague sense that there may be some confidence trouble, it is easier to keep plodding forward to the ways that feel easy and habitual.

This last item expresses my particular flavor: avoidance.

For most of my life I never really questioned my confidence. This is not because it was flooding out of me like an unchecked fire hydrant, but more because I had never thought to ask. Think more of a head-in-the-sand ostrich than a prancing peacock. But the thing about denial is that it works wonders until it doesn't.

Often, we take just enough risks in life to feel comfy, to not rock the boat or stray too far from the easiest, straightforward path in front of us. This is a kind of fear that disguises itself as predictability and routine. I had just enough confidence to leapfrog from rock to rock but only if the waters around me were even-tempered and accommodating.

It is this situational confidence that is the trickster. It rocks us on gossamer wings, gently suspending us aloft one minute and then dropping us on the cold, hard ground the next. We barely realize that we are in a constant state of just scarcely getting by.

But true confidence is not person- or place-dependent, it is not about feeling beautiful only if someone else tells us so. It is not about pats on the back, piles of gold stars, or accumulating thousands of "likes." It is a different creature entirely. The closest that I can get to it is in more references to the Earth—a confidence with broad and tenacious roots, like the presence of a tree centuries old.

Why, despite all of our advances in income, in job titles, in opportunities in the last century, does confidence continue to be an Achilles' heel for women? What is the persistent, repetitive messaging, from both our cultural and familial indoctrinations, that sustains an epidemic of inner distrust and lack of self-esteem?

Why do so many women seem to struggle with confidence, entangled in the messy vitriol of self-sabotage, hate, and doubt? I never realized what a sticky question this was, with its many layers and layers of complication. What is happening in our early training that shows up so persistently later in womanhood?

Invisibility

Arriving at the intersection of this questioning, we are greeted with the complexities of individual life experiences, family pressures, cultural and racial impacts, all influencing the many reasons women struggle to feel seen and heard. There are so many factors hidden behind why women have trouble feeling okay taking up their own physical and psychic space.

Are we or are we not "making progress" as women in this world? In most work arenas empowerment appears to be taking hold. Women have a layer of armor that makes them seem poised and positive. Occasionally, our softer selves are allowed to shine beyond our tough exteriors. But what is still happening under that protective shell? Do true feelings of confidence lie within our velvet underbellies—in the unlit passages of women's psyches, places where we are potentially more vulnerable, but honest?

It is within the deep psyche that we find a graveyard of *little things* that diminish our confidence. This silent burial place holds an accumulation of all our unexamined, repressed experiences and feelings, most of which are the results of the subtle inequity we have faced for being female in a male-dominated world.

Blatant discrimination loudly persists despite the legal and financial progress women have made. Even so, it is the repetitive layering of little things that work on us more cleverly. Showing up in brief interactions or in smooth power grabs, they are ubiquitous and difficult to catch right in the moment. Microtraumas might come in "innocently" ignorant comments dropped, leaving a sulfurous scent lingering in the air. Or they may come in eyeballs hovering, lurking, and penetrating our clothes with a coyote's drooling smirk.

These sneaky little things make us doubt ourselves, make us hesitate, make us slow to react. Sometimes there is the shock of disbelief after an incident of inequity or harassment.

Sometimes the fear of confrontation.

Or a longing not to make a fuss.

And so, we feel confused, reduced, ashamed, and this all layers us in invisibility.

In or outside of the workplace, women are constantly managing the buildup of these little things. A hand placed on a butt or thigh. The leaning in with the door closed. The threat of what could be.

Most women have at least one, if not a handful, of stories of incidents that made them feel small or threatened, which often occurred at times or in places that they least expected it. One memory forces itself forward in my mind, a time when I was a tired, road-worn student driving home from college. The highways were full for the holidays so it took me a little while to perceive a car alongside me, pacing my exact speed along the road. There was a moment of intuition, something suspicious about the other vehicle as it tried to keep moving with me. Looking over, the driver had his penis out. He was greedily masturbating, hoping for some reaction.

Such a little thing, the surprise of a randomly exposed highway penis. But what is really at work here? The flexing of pathological power, to push yourself on someone else even if it is only in mind games. I knew I was safe in my car, but there were feelings that lingered afterward: a flip of the stomach, the gnawing of my insides. A vague anxiety or a creepy feeling that chases us long after a moment in which our boundaries have been trampled. The impact of these microaggressions, which are like tiny notes of confidence-killing dialogue written into the script of our lives, grinds on us willfully over the years.

These subtle teachings in invisibility show up in what is taught to us through our family lineage. They live on in us through the life experiences of those that came before us, those that are never very far away. The lives of our grandmothers softly exist in us somewhere still. Our matrilineal lines continue on like nested Russian dolls, our cells having lived within our mother's womb, which lived in her mother's womb.

These subtleties show up in what is shared. Brutal violence and glaring injustices toward women are taking place somewhere on this planet *right now, in this very moment*. We feel ourselves connected, woven together as women, our communal hair creating a tremendous braid of different colors and textures. That despite all of our efforts to compartmentalize and make separate, our hearts are bound still.

These subtleties show up in what is felt. Everyday safety, or a lack thereof, acts as a looming stressor, keeping women just a little more rigid and suspicious in their skins. Like walking the path of our lives with our shoelaces tied together; everything is just a little bit harder. Awkwardly hopping instead of confidently gliding, women do not even realize the full physical and energetic burden that this feeling of uncertain safety brings.

These subtleties show up in what is sensed. When we slow and listen, we can perceive how the patriarchy is entrenched in our thought patterns and world view. The fossil-like structures, systems, governments, religions, and industries that have created the scaffolding of our culture continue to struggle with making space for the presence and voices of women. Or blatantly, outrightly still treat women as subordinate, second-class citizens. Author Anand Giridharadas wonders, "How might war and capitalism and criminal justice and a thousand other things be different had they not been designed with half of humanity locked outside the door?"[3]

What a tremendous, painful deficit this has created.

And we hesitate to step forward still.

Although our stories of how and where it happens may be different, most women are familiar with the experience of becoming translucent, as if we are overlaid in clear ink. This sensation is to look down at your hands, at your torso, at your feet and to feel yourself becoming more and more faint. Even now, in the twenty-first century, the pain of disregard still lingers in the subtle contours of the female mind.

When a persistent feeling of translucence sets in, it lays a plastic film, a false barrier along the lens of your self-perception. With every passing interaction that makes you feel unseen and unheard, you begin to believe that there may be nothing worth seeing about you. Many women remain as invisible to themselves as they are to the rest of the world.

We must come to know ourselves in full color. Our freedom demands we paint in sparkly metallics and watercolor blotches and allow ourselves the smushy forgivingness of oil paints. Let us be willing to be seen, if by no one else than by ourselves. And to see more clearly what continually influences our confidence—raising or lowering it by turns.

Myths of Confidence

Our society's commonly held beliefs are more like gas than matter. Tiny, invisible particles surround us entirely, constantly. They have no fixed shape or volume or odor, but they are always there, being breathed into our lungs and transported through our veins. It is the sneaky, imperceptible influence of these particles of belief that allows them to live on in the deep, unconscious vaults of our minds.

Fortunately, with effort, questioning, and occasional sudden shocks of insight, we can awaken to their presence, turn on a fan, and blow them out the window. We can refuse to breathe them into the recesses of our lungs. When we begin to pay closer attention to the reasons why we feel such a lack of confidence, we start to perceive the myths and unhelpful stories we were bought into. And we can then replace those stories with something that rings with truth.

But how do we know what's true when the word *confidence* is thrown far and wide with all sorts of varied usages? We clearly need this thing called confidence, but it doesn't always seem obvious as to what it is exactly, or how to get it.

Most often confidence is described or insinuated to be something that exists outside of us, like something to be gathered up through self-betterment, power poses, and impressions created for other people. Confidence becomes a list of attributes that we feel we have to pack ourselves with, a polyester filler to be stuffed into our innards, making us appear bigger than we feel. But the inherent flaw with all of this fake-it-till-you-make-it business is that faking implies that from the very get go you don't actually have what you need.

Deconstructing the myths of confidence helps us understand all of these surface scratching ideas we hold within our culture and how many of them are based in a sense of lack. That we are fundamentally missing something. When we expand our thinking and make space for all that we contain, we may start to see how widening our sphere of self-acceptance lets in room for fear, doubt, and honesty—or that we can change the rules on this thing called confidence. Perhaps true confidence is less about being untouchable or unstoppable and more about acknowledging our uncomfortable vulnerabilities, acknowledging their purpose, becoming softer and more available in the process.

Extroverted = Confidence?

When I was a child the term *shy strong* had yet to be invented. Lists of powerful, innovative introverts did not exist on the internet. Quiet people were yet to be perceived as having special superpowers. Instead, introversion was linked to some sense of deep defectiveness, a fundamental weakness of character.

Being a serious, watchful child, on some level I perceived myself as a few handholds away from confident. In a deep crevice of my mind, confidence was a special state reserved for professional soccer players and businesswomen in long, important meetings. Perhaps a few dictators at its worst.

I was plagued by the influence of one of western society's most clingy and prevailing myths: *You must be extroverted to be confident.*

Writer Susan Cain calls this the "Extrovert Ideal—the omnipresent belief that the ideal self is gregarious, alpha, and comfortable in the spotlight. The archetypal extrovert prefers action to contemplation, risk-taking to heed-taking, certainty to doubt . . . Introverts living under the Extrovert Ideal are like women living in a man's world, discounted because of a trait that goes to the core of who they are."[4]

Women are not necessarily introverted. But this notion of extroverted confidence has a masculine undertone to it. There is an assumed extroverted quality to the confidence paradigm that has been dominant in our society.

Where does confidence live outside the bounds of our cultural expectations of being social, charming, a bit breezy? There are so many women who actually show up with genuine self-trust in their lives, but they don't allow themselves to identify as confident because they don't associate with extroversion.

I notice this in so many of the quiet, sensitive ones around me. They are not interested in tearing up the dance floor, dominating the room with conversation, or taking pictures of their dinner and posting it on Instagram. It doesn't even occur to them.

No, they are not snobby, stuck up, or antisocial.

Theirs is a quieter presence. They are the observers, the listeners of the world.

Not to be underestimated.

The reservoirs of an introvert's strength can run deep, but they just don't feel the need to splash you in the face with it.

Our cultural expectation of extroversion being better than introversion is so enveloping that we are quick to slide right over the standing of an introvert. We orient with the hulking assumption that extroversion and confidence are the same beast so readily that we push right past the beautiful intelligence or special insights of the introverted female. Still.

But at its core, confidence does not care about rigid definitions of introverts or extroverts. Frequently used and enduringly contentious, you may decide to throw these terms or categories out entirely. Because we are just so quick to seal ourselves in orderly cubby holes, we miss our unique expression on the introvert/extrovert spectrum.

The truth is that we exist within a continuum of experience as humans. You can be shy courageous or quiet strong or nice tough. It is accepting and loving ourselves fully that is a true act of confidence.

I am reminded that confidence has room for the internal complexity of a woman and her great ranges of experience and expression. When we trust in ourselves, we feel how seemingly perfect compartments of black and white don't exist and that we are more like charcoal art, roaming obsidian and smudgy silvers, elaborate blends and layers of our own free creation.

This leads us to our next confidence misconception.

No Fear = Confidence?

If you are confident, you will never feel afraid.

Let me be clear.

Confidence does not mean the absence of fear. But somehow in the midst of putting on our emotional coat of armor to get by in the world and come home safely at night, there are those of us who have convinced ourselves that truly confident people are never afraid. We believe that fear is weakness and the vulnerability that accompanies it is to be avoided at all costs.

This false idea is sold to us by advertisers too. It is so easy to want to aspire to their messages. We read books, see posts, find articles that endlessly mix the word *unafraid* with *bold, fierce, daring.* We buy into this belief that every molecule of our fear can be banished forever with some secret formula or listicle of overly simplistic suggestions. "Be a fearless woman, fearless entrepreneur, fearless leader," they say.

And we want this, right? Because who wouldn't want to be free of the discomfort, the murky confusion, the hot agitation that fear can bring?

But it is our relationship with fear that is at the crux here. Can we let fear flow through us in its naturalness, accepting its presence? Because the truth is that when we are right up against that edge, when we take a moment to look down and see how far up we've actually come, how high of a mountain we have climbed, of course we are going to feel nervous. Anxious. Shaky even. Fear does not leave us in acts of fearlessness.

I am not going to tell you just to transmute your fear into excitement. If you can do this, great. But if your fear is some immovable, megalithic slab, then stop. Stop trying to slam yourself into that thing to get it to move.

Stop your running starts.

Stop bashing yourself against it, over and over again.

Just let the fear be.

Fear is a normal, intelligent response to doing something different, new, or unknown. It is our most base, prehistoric emotion and there is no way you are going to exile it from your human experience. So, stop using it as an excuse not to trust yourself.

The truth is that we want our confidence to shimmy its way easily to us. We want whatever we try, dream, create, or risk to fall into our laps like an eager, slobbery puppy. Without fear and on the first try if you please.

And there is a certain confidence to be gained from things going our way, for sure. This is to feel a sense of gratification for hard efforts put forth, receiving confirmation of our sweat and toil. To hold our trophies up high, pump our fists in the air, and feel truly exceptional.

But then there is a different kind of confidence altogether, the type that arises when things don't go our way. The kind that exists when we are still giving it our all and we see nothing come of it. No acknowledgment, no fancy awards, no praise. Just crickets.

This is the confidence that actually comes from your lowest of lows, from feelings of failure, maybe even rejection. It is the confidence that comes from getting dragged through the mud or having the wind taken out of your sails, all ambitions sent adrift. The kind that is mired in the most overwhelming, unbelievable, ugly fear. It is the confidence that comes when we let it break us, pulverize us, change us, leaving no other option than to be deeply affected, maybe even permanently altered.

We may finally be convinced to surrender instead of trying harder.

We may graciously allow ourselves to wear our real face, with its swollen, tear-lined, red eyes, instead of putting on the usual happy mask.

Because the heart of this fear wants us to better understand what our confidence truly rests on. We may realize now that our fragile self-trust was oriented, even unconsciously, from the power given by others. We may see how the slightest bumps in the road shake us to our core, tight fingers grasping for reassurance. That our confidence was really a tree trunk secretly rotted, easily cracked, and ready to be blown over.

Testing the strength within your roots, you may more clearly perceive what authentic confidence means to you. You may understand that in these stormy, fear-ridden times, your inner resources have been expanding below the surface. That there is some new reservoir of grit, resiliency, inner knowing, and unconditional self-love that has been flowing, fed in the dark.

This kind of confidence softens us, lightens our load, forgives us when we are not feeling brave. It takes an entirely different approach, not doing battle with fear but instead taking hold of its wrinkled, ancient hand. Looking it deep in the eyes, we can feel fear's primal intelligence trying to protect us from hurt. And we can say, "Oh dear, fear, thank you for trying to keep me safe. I witness you." Acknowledging its presence alongside us, we may decide to stop giving our power away to fear. We may conclude that we no longer want to feed it so much of our time and energy, letting it grow bigger than it needs to be.

Moving forward and feeling fear next to us, we can use it to belong to ourselves more fully, coming back to self-trust over and over again.

No Doubt = Confidence?

Our next myth likes to come right on the heels of fear. Here it is.

If you are confident, you will never doubt yourself.

Self-doubt feels like a childhood friend to fear. The clutch of self-doubt will paralyze us if we let it. We long to move forward but we don't think we can. We pace, we strain at our tether, we run ourselves in ragged circles like a dog on a shortened leash.

There are so many versions to our self-doubting. There is the doubt of comparisons, the nagging, insecure voices that tell us that someone else is already doing it better. Then there is the doubt of not being ready, convincing ourselves that we need more teachers, more time, more training, more of *something* in order to move forward. There is also the sneaky, persistent type of doubt that wants to protect us from pain—the stop-before-we-start version.

Society preaches some slick version of confidence to us in all sorts of ways: podcasts, slogans, wall art, and Instagram blurbs. A skin of confidence made easy to slip on, right? This makes us believe that we have to have our self-doubt all orderly and nicely-behaved before we can take action.

We find so many ways to stay put. We think we couldn't possibly start that exercise class because we are already so out-of-shape. Or we couldn't think to start teaching that poetry class because our life is not yet perfectly managed, the kids keep waking us up at night and we are still getting gray hairs. Still.

This is sort of like being a bird and expecting to learn how to fly on the first try. But no bird learns how to fly on its first go around. Not one. How do they learn? By practice, by the reinforcement of their parents, by *trying*. Granted there is a nonnegotiable biological impulse pushing them along, but birds learn to fly in the doing.

And this is the thing about confidence that we bungle up. We think it is supposed to come in the beginning, that we need it for the starting. We think it is the prerequisite to action, some mysterious igniting force. But we have a serious flaw in our expectation and understanding of how this sequence really works.

Confidence arrives in the end, not the beginning. It magnifies in the doingness, in the tryingness, in the one-foot-placed-in-front-of-the-otherness, or sometimes even in the falling-flat-on-your-faceness.

Hey, you could just continue to wait it out.

But the truth is that your confidence may never really kick in the way you want it to. Never. Ever.

You will still be waiting, working deep grooves in the ground with all of your walking back and forth, your collar yanked tight.

Because when exactly is your life going to feel perfectly behaved?

When will it feel nicely contained?

When will it be entirely safe to proceed?

Can you be confident enough to allow for natural periods of doubt, the occasional confidence impasse that can hit anyone at any time? It may show up as a divorce, a death, the loss of a job, or a misguided business endeavor. A rejection, an ending, a period of grief.

Something that forces you to come to a grinding stop.

Something that makes everything in your life, all the tedious minutia, suddenly feel very untethered, floating in midair.

Those experiences are opportunities to reassess your motivations and direction.

"What the hell have you been doing anyway?" they ask you.

Self-doubt is an experience that brings us closer to our edge, closer to the marrow of what really matters. It pauses us, pushes us around in the dark corners for a while, and then sends us back into our lives, maybe a little jangly around the edges but awake, much more aware and on our toes.

When life is causing you to reassess, it is what you *do* with your confidence crisis, your period of doubt, that matters. Will you let it teach you? Will you listen to the deeper whisperings of the doubt to grow something different in yourself? Are you brave enough to feel paper-thin for a while without changing or masking the experience?

What if doubt has been a friend instead of a foe all along?

If just for today, welcome your self-doubt with open arms. Don't try to smother it in platitudes of false confidence or read it cheesy wall art. Don't do anything with it, other than let it be real and true.

Confidence Hunting

Returning to the energy of the naturally confident owl at the beginning of this chapter, we are reminded of a more instinctual trust. Channeling the owl's tremendous ability to perceive in the dark, it is time for you to more clearly see the many different examples of confidence around you. Enhancing the scope of your perspective allows you to see in ways others don't, sensing the truth behind veils of illusion or manipulation.

You may begin to notice that some of the people you identify as being confident are not necessarily the most competent or even pleasant to be around. What does toxic high confidence look like? It can show up with socially inappropriate, aggressive, argumentative, uninhibited, or unempathetic behavior. You may come to sense how often hyperinflated confidence is just a mask for insecurity or fear.

And what about more sexy versions of confidence that may try to distract and coerce you? With an owl's sight you may begin to sensitively perceive all of the confidence distortions, even the overly spiritualized, pleasing but deeply false kinds. Like the woman with all of the beautiful white gauzy dresses, long feather earrings, and arm tattoos meditating over some gorgeous rocky expanse. This is the other extreme, the woman who has it all figured out every moment of the day, robes flowing, and perfectly at ease. She is a glossy seductress.

With a perch at the highest reaches of the tree line, wings growing beneath your shirt, what will this owl vision reveal to you? Confidence hunting allows you to better understand what more healthy, grounded versions of self-trust feel like to you.

Instructions and Invitations

Good questions have this way of working on us. Because in the chaos and confusion of modern overstimulation, it is not always easy to know what we hold essential. Take the time now to wrestle, tango, even fly with these questions until some truth pours out of you.

Before proceeding any further with these inquiries, I encourage you to have a fresh space like a new journal that exists solely for this purpose. These questions and their answers need a home. I see your journal and this book living next to each other, enjoying the pressing comfort of each other's weight.

It is in this purposeful asking that you will be creating a practice of self-care and discovery. I want the words you are reading on the page to move from your eyeballs and your brain into a felt experience, soaking it deep into your body.

Your inner knowing is not sourced from conceptual philosophies, but instead comes through the power of your lived experience. By becoming more human, not less. It is not enough to contemplate these pages quickly and passively as a bystander on the sidelines. Make this your own.

It is true that when you are first starting, a blank, milky page can be terribly intimidating, Sometimes, when I am lost with where to begin, I start with columns of simple, individual words. Flipping through old journals, often I find pages of lists filled with words that are beautiful or uncommon, words that delight me, like *sibilance* and *interstice* and *pendulous*. I could get lost in strange word combinations, the imaginings of what *livid magenta* or a *velvet umbra* might look like. I can get punch-drunk on the witchery of words.

But perhaps word crafting is not for you. A journaling practice is assessible for most, but perhaps you would like to paint out these inquiries instead. Maybe you feel wisdom comes to you in color tones and textures. I love that.

Whatever your creative process may be, let it be one that moves you out of your analyzing, logical self and allows you to flow with whatever wants to emerge—no matter how strange, shocking, or silly. Follow what has energy to you and makes you feel alive.

Take your time with these exercises and practices. Chew slowly. Integrate intentionally. Grow patience with what information wants to arise from you. The creative process inherently asks you to connect with your confidence. It asks you to trust in yourself with no guarantees around outcome or result. It asks you to sink back into honesty, humility, and compassion with whatever wants to arise out of you in that moment.

Cracking your new journal open to the unknown of a fresh page, let's spiral back to some of the questions at the beginning of this chapter:

What has drawn you to these confidence inquiries?

How do you view your confidence in your life right now?

You could take some time to answer these questions directly, or you could write the word CONFIDENCE in large letters at the top of your page and free write for ten minutes. Just hold space in free flow about anything and everything that comes to mind when you think about the word *confidence*. Unleash a river of words. Move your hand across the page. You don't need to edit or censor yourself. There is no screwing this up.

It is often in the awkward pauses of our writing flow that we can sweep the hidden corners of our mind, suddenly surprised by what wants to surface. Don't let any moments of rest or vacillation stop you, for it is in these little hesitations, when we think we can go no further, that interesting insights arise. Try to write for the full ten minutes.

Here are a few more writing invitations to consider if you would like to explore further:

- *Honestly examining the influences of your cultural "soup," what are some of the myths that you have believed about confidence? How do these influences rub up against and oppose your current truths?*

- *Think now to your family line, even beyond your parents. What did your elders teach you (or not teach you) about confidence in their spoken words, in their actions, in their hidden messaging, in their body language?*

- *In her book* Power and Sex, *three-time Noble Peace Prize nominee Scilla Elworthy, Ph.D., describes what a woman looks like in her complete, embodied power: "People feel safe with her because she has her feet planted within the earth."⁵ This is a woman who has shot her roots downward and is clear about where she receives her nourishment. Vertical roots. Horizontal roots. Roots that touch the roots of others. Considering this definition, what makes you feel most rooted?*

CHAPTER THREE

Sovereign Natives

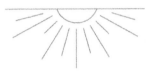

"With every new breath she created a new matrix for herself.
And when She was done,
She looked around and found Herself in a sea of sisters.
Who this whole time, had been doing the exact same thing."[1]
—REBECCA CAMPBELL

Again and again she raises her curved head to smash down on the rocks of the stoic cliffs, crushing, sliding, and obstinately creeping through them. They are no match for this hardheaded storm of a sea. Exquisite and treacherous all at once, she lives in one continuous rhythm of in and out, contraction and release. I watch the slow grin of her mouth, the gnawing, almost-breaking waves falling forward invitingly, only to coyly pull away again. I feel all the time with her in these doings, the transitory tides, the insistence of erosion, and the unavoidability of change. The flow of this mischievous vixen lingers in me, drenching me in a memory of my own naturalness.

Flying Revolutionaries

The ocean is a teacher in the movement of friction. Friction is the vibration of resistance created when one object moves against another. An ignition of flint scraped across smooth steel. The texture of two books sliding against each other as they find their place on the shelf. The feeling of heat when your own two hands touch, rubbing against each other by the fire.

There is also friction created when we live or act in ways that scrape against the societal yardsticks.

This kind of friction is often spectacularly defiant and rebellious.

What better way is there to illustrate and teach us about the theme of resistance than through the ancient stories of the fierce feminine? In these stories, we see lives lived outside a culture rigid in patriarchal values—a time when we lived as if we knew the Earth and the sea as our mothers.

Back when God was a woman.

I close my eyes and try to imagine the feral spirits of these unrestrained prehistoric women, wild, long hair and calluses on their feet. I dream of them as sovereign over their bodies, their passions, their creativity, their land, but some quiet part of me questions even this. It is hard to truly know what life was like for these long-ago women.

We are left breathing life into them with the bits and pieces that we have, using biographies of the many styles of the untamed woman as hope. Knowing, singing, and repeating their myths can feed us as modern women. Swallowing their stories deep into our bellies is a sometimes forgotten nourishment in our male-dominated epoch.

Psychologist and storyteller Sharon Blackie describes the importance of story when she says:

Stories matter, you see. They're not just entertainment—stories matter because humans are narrative creatures. . . . It's a function of our biology, the way our brains have evolved over time. We make sense of the world and fashion our identities through the sharing and passing of stories. And so the stories that we tell ourselves about the world and our place in it, and the stories that are told to us by others about the world and our place in it, shape not just our own lives, but the world around us. The cultural narrative is the culture.[2]

Knowing now the undeniable power of stories, what exactly have we been telling ourselves?

Judeo-Christian cosmology infected western civilization with the idea that the female body and female sexuality is the downfall of *man*kind. We know we are in trouble when the predominating modern story of the first woman is based on being formed from a "defective rib of man's breast, which was bent contrary to him, and so therefore it is in woman's nature to deceive."[3] Because she dared to eat the fruit of the Tree of Knowledge, Eve became the scapegoat for all of humanity's suffering. She and her man were kicked out of this garden paradise—ostracized and shamed. In a final act of punishment, women were declared by God to be forever subservient to men, having been determined weak and faithless.

The cultural underpinnings from the story of Eve in the biblical book of Genesis have supplied us with very clear messaging for the last many thousands of years: that women are subordinate and problematic. They're not to be trusted by themselves or others.

If this is what we tell ourselves, this is what shapes us.

But when we look back to the time beyond and before Eve, we discover rich examples of a very different type of story. In her book *Women Who Fly*, anthropologist Serinity Young homes in on myths from around the world of sky-going women, a particularly fascinating subset of powerful females that includes witches, mystics, angels, demons, and fairies. These women (and feminine spirits) were provocative enough to transcend gravity, so potent that even the rules of physics could not pin them down.

Many of the airborne women depicted in these myths defied the traditional ideas of the female as nurturing and receptive, breasts ready for a mouth. Instead, they made space for the great expanse of feminine experience and expression. Young explains:

> *Flying females from a wide variety of cultures are linked to sexuality, death and rebirth, or immortality. In different places and historical periods, there were remarkably similar discourses about the unpredictable powers of aerial women, who could be generous or withholding, empowering or destructive. Because of their uncertain nature, the question arose as to how they could be controlled: whether by supplication or coercion. Over time they flew through a universe of ever-increasing constraint in which similar means were used to capture and domesticate them, to turn them into handmaidens of male desire and ambition.*[4]

These flying revolutionaries are a particular curiosity to me, the way they have full trust in their wings. I want to fly with them, to shapeshift, to be uncontained. I long for their sight, the skilled reach of their eyes to pull in great vistas and wandering ranges. I wonder how it would feel to call the sky home, to be that much closer to the vault of the heavens and its vast canopy of stars.

But while I enjoy dreaming of the lightness in their bones and the pleasurable tension in the full stretch of their wings, I would balk at actually emulating their magical flight.

It remains a lovely vision, but the truth is: I am terrified of flying.

This terror started late one night on my final red-eye home with a feeling of the seat giving way beneath me. After a series of very long international flights at the tender age of twenty, I had my first panic attack on a plane.

What if I never reach home again? became an unrelenting loop in my head, masterminded by some manic inner DJ. The firmness of the chair, the floor, the childlike trust that kept that chunk of metal in the air up until that time—*poof*—they evaporated.

Fear can be such a fool. I know the numbers, the stats, the facts about the much higher likelihood of dying in a car accident than on a plane. But when survival fear lodges in you like a pesky burr, the rational mind becomes like an incompetent pair of tweezers, unable to evict that embedded terror.

I will save you the last twenty years' worth of all the things I have tried to pluck this fear out of me. I decided long ago not to let this stubborn trembling, this cool slick of sweat, this thrashing heart, ground me. I will not let it stop me from living.

And I see no irony in the fact that, despite my fear of flying, I've also developed a marked kinship to those who live to fly. I am in constant communication with my feathered friends, the ones who never question flying. Among them:

- The bald eagle that glides the airstream ten feet above me, our pathways casually intersecting.
- The pair of osprey that circle the great sequoia in the backyard, their bodies apparently blending and merging kaleidoscopically as they go round and round.
- The glossy raven lovers, melodramatic and urgent, calling to each other while my sneakered feet caress the forest path.
- The demure herons shimmering and softly dancing in the light of the waves.
- The hummingbird, green breast glistening, spiraling in its flower hunt.
- The Cooper's hawk, an undisturbed statue, sitting, just watching, from the back fence.

- The barred owl, just five feet from me, our eyes level, penetrating me with its black scowl, grazing the depth of my soul, before flying to its mate.

Lately it has been the western screech owl that has been calling. It has been singing to me every night that the windows are still open and from out of the obsidian depths of the forest beyond our backyard, its call is a series of eerie, trilled notes, sounding half-animal, half-strange spirit. I wonder what other creature could make that sound—it seems to live between two worlds.

Me and the winged ones are family in a way. Because I am also feeling between worlds, stories, lives.

Birds have always been symbols of transcendence, living somewhere between heaven and earth. They are thought to be messengers to the divine, traversing the containment of our world to breach the sky and touch the soul in their ecstatic flight. And I take it as no coincidence that I feel such a closeness to these mysterious beauties. I admire how easily they trust their wings to perform their duty.

They teach me about letting go and abandoning control—control over myself and control over my world.

They teach me about sweeping and soaring as I please, the freedom of choosing adventure over fear.

And they show me the privilege of being unrestrained, independent, and fully alive, invigorated by the force of the wind through my hair. I can be challenged and live through it. I can place my fear in a brave nest and just let it rest there.

The stories of the winged-women, the sky-sailing wild ones, pique my curiosity. I want to gather the spirit of these stories within myself, the essence of these creatures who dared, and then learn from them. From the beautiful apsaras of Hindu myth to the swan maidens of European fairy tales, the Valkyries of Norse legend, and the winged

Greek goddesses Iris and Nike we may discover an internal fascination with the many expressions of female power and sexuality.

This includes tales of the dangerous ones, figures of terror such as the Furies, witches, and wild women, like Lilith and Morgan le Fay. They all knew how to create friction. These stories bring us to the brink of experience, to hold the potential for blessings and curses and everything in between.

Quietening now, think back to your stories. What tales have been whispered in your ear, and where do you store them? What did you take on as your own?

There was no *Strong Is the New Pretty* or *Good Night Stories for Rebel Girls* when I was a young girl, however I am grateful for the emergence and growing desire for books like this in the marketplace. These books are not just for the young women that they will influence, but also for the parents—especially mothers—reading them aloud. These new stories are a lifeline, planting seeds of possibility within our collective consciousness, like an updraft of potential for all young women seeing and dreaming this fresh paradigm into being.

Subversive Sentries

Ideas of femininity surround us, but the actual experience or embodiment of the wild feminine is rarer. What if we actively worked and engaged with a support team of feminine archetypes that illuminate the healthy, strong feminine?

This is to call consciously upon a crew of feminine confidence archetypes, a gathering of what I like to call the *sentries*. These four archetypes are all boldly feminine, while at the same time easily embody a unity of the masculine and feminine energy in us all. And each of these archetypal energies has its own unique expression of a deeply rooted sense of confidence.

- *The Space Dancer (the Dakini principle):* She has the voice of the revolution.
- *The Inner Healer (our self-healing principle):* She has the voice of bone-knowing.
- *Wild Gaia (the ancient Earth mama):* She has the voice of your soul-root.
- *The Artist-Visionary (the midwife of creative experience):* She sparks imagination and encourages us to express our true nature.

We will be using these archetypes not as something to harshly compare ourselves to or as another pedestal to tumble down from. We will look to these beauties to set the tone, to encourage us, and to offer guidance as we step bravely into our own storms.

They help us to remember that we are not alone.

But let's not humanize these energies. We are less likely to encase them in our own personal dramas and stories when we can work with them as more of an *essence*. These energies are examples and guides that we all have the potential to know and uncover within ourselves. Take whatever wisdom they have to offer, as it best syncs with you.

I introduce these archetypal ideas now so that we can let their energy infuse all our future questioning and time together. These models are meant to be loving and impartial, but interactive, showing up just when you need them. We will also use writing invitations after the introduction of each archetype as an opportunity for us to connect with each one more intimately.

Call in the Space Dancer

It is an image forever imprinted in my mind, like a postcard that will never wrinkle. In this picture there is pasture and farmland painted in sleepy pinks, grays, and blues, the colors dampened to a softer hue as if they had been wiped over by a moist cloth. Halos of flies hover around the grazing horses and their tails swish, their muscles shiver automatically, like even this exertion is without effort. The only sound seems to be from the land spirits humming, the subtlest of vibration being released from the earth. The air is weighted with the most ineffable peace, a reachable, touchable grace.

I traveled to this undisturbed place for the very specific reason of going inside. Returning to this memory, I am twenty years old and accompanied by a group of students as part of the School for International Training's Tibetan Studies Program. We are slowly making our way through northern India, Nepal, and Tibet; and on this day, we are completely off the beaten path in Tibet, discovering destroyed or rundown monasteries. So here, *going inside* refers to going inside ourselves, going inside the land, and going inside the rubble that is left.

Many of these precious places look like a pile of old rocks from the outside. But when you go in, you find the most indescribable treasures, mostly in the form of ancient artwork. There are paintings that span the floor and ceiling. Much of this art is covered in soot from burning butter lamps, or simply from the ash and dirt of years gone by. Some are even pockmarked with bullet holes from the time of the Chinese Cultural Revolution. But then there are others, loved and preserved, gleaming with care and tenderly sheltered from harm. In these magical places, I felt a palpable presence emanating from all of the past and present spiritual practice.

On this particular day we were visiting the Ralung Gompa Monastery, which was founded in 1180 C.E. and had once housed 30,000 monks. As we began wandering through the outer hallway, we took in the great detail on the painted statues of the protective deities and the ornate patterning of the hand-painted borders running along the edges of each room.

Just as we reached the outskirts of the main shrine room, there was a murmur rising among the guides. Then a long, tense pause . . .

And then the women of the group were promptly led outside.

It all happened too fast to protest. "What happened?" I wondered aloud into open air. The best translation that could be given was that we were considered "unclean."

From what I can remember of that moment, there was a bit of a shock, but nothing that lingered for too long. When you are a guest of another culture, you quickly learn to roll with almost anything. And of course, this was not my first brush with sexism.

But there was still some outrage, mostly with a feeling that there was some gap of misunderstanding. *I'm not unclean!* rolled the protest in my head.

And yet, there was another voice there too, reminding me that *I am a dirty woman.*

I don't know if any of the women within the group were actually bleeding at that moment, but clearly it did not matter. It was even just the *potential* for bleeding that was punishable. Dangerous.

Instead of recognizing menstrual blood as the rich food from which all human life grows, our monthly bleeding during our years of fertility is considered taboo and nasty.

Instead of seeing the way the uterus cleanses itself each month as miraculous, women are taught to hide and sanitize this natural process within themselves.

Instead of considering a woman at her bleeding time to be so clean that there is a force of spiritual purity that moves through her, women are taught a weighted shame.

Sacred turned polluted.

We are all dirty women.

There is a powerful, persistent fear of women's bodies that is not unique to my experience, but that lives across many cultures and countries. Just as there can be so many different interpretations of a woman's bleeding time, there remain many clashing views on the role of women and the practice of Buddhism. In old, orthodox circles there still exists an idea that being born in female form prevents women from attaining realization at all.

Despite its lack of support, there is a rogue vein of female subversion that runs through Tibetan Buddhism. According to the ancient Indian language of Sanskrit, the female embodiment of enlightenment is called a *dakini*. The Tibetan word for dakini, or *khandro*, translates as "sky goer" or "space dancer." Traditionally, a dakini would be a kickass female practitioner, usually a consort of a great master, who could express the enlightened female principle of nonduality, which transcends gender altogether.

Dakinis possess the awakened quality of leaving the solidness of the ground to go play in either the vastness of open sky or the open mind. They are said to be able to help us break through obstacles in our thinking, destroying ignorance without hesitation, surprising us with their suddenly fierce energy.

The Space Dancer is unafraid of being complex and contradictory. She can be sensual, frisky, and enticing. But don't get too comfortable. In the next instant, she might swing her curved knife at you, cutting through your ego attachment without warning. She could lovingly hold you with the compassion of a great mother for one moment and then flash her wild vagina at you in the next. A dakini could be a living woman, but within a deeper level of meaning, she could be a "luminous, subtle, spiritual energy, the key, the gatekeeper, the guardian of the unconditioned state . . . sometimes dakinis appear as messengers, sometimes as guides, and sometimes as protectors."

We can connect with dakinis through ancient stories, through living spiritual teachers, or more importantly, as an essence that we all contain. I often call on the spirit of the Space Dancer that lives inside me when I am being asked to move outside my sphere of comfort. She helps us find our most shaky stretch. But there is also something completely holy in what is hardest for us. She expertly knows how to model a state of groundlessness and she easily cuts through some of our most maligning patterns, such as shame, self-doubt, and fear of change.

On a solo hike in Colorado this past summer, I was awakened from the monotonous, dry mastication of gravel under my shoes—*crunch, crunch, crunch*— with some sharp jab of an invitation from the Space Dancer to climb. Already whirling with the effects of high altitude, I had the sudden urge—no compulsion—to strive to reach the highest point.

Straining my neck skyward, I could see a very steep mass of boulders, like an oversized pile that some she-god had thrown together in a hasty attempt to clean up. It felt like a place where the dakinis might play. The first of many shy cairns aided me with a general sense of direction and with tar-like lumps in my throat and belly, one foot seemed to follow another into the land of the Space Dancer.

Halfway up, I made a pit stop for some temporary hyperventilating, and clinging to the rock like a desperate baby monkey, I managed not to look down (too much). I still could not clearly identify what was drawing me forward.

Was there something I needed to prove?

Was there something I needed to learn?

One foothold at a time, one handhold at a time finally brought me to the thinner air. Despite its breathtaking beauty, it felt hard to engage my full senses. I can't remember what I heard, what I smelled. Even though that rock pile had probably been resting there for hundreds of years, sitting on the very top edge made me feel like a feather precariously placed on a dissolving sandcastle. There was nothing solid about it. Looking out over a vast mountain range and a drop thousands of feet down, against every message my body wanted to give me, I forced myself to stay. To stay with the liquid, scorching panic seizing my heart and chest, the adrenaline of instinctual fear, demanding, pushing, compressing all my soft parts.

I sat there clutching my rock, frozen.

"Just stay, just stay, just stay, just stay . . ." were the circular and persistent words on my tongue. A labyrinth of soothing tones. Perhaps the dakinis had called me there, but their lessons were not ones of bliss and fluff. No spiritual rapture here.

This was my fear of death openly tenderizing me.

Stripping my pretense bare.

Evaporating the will of my personality.

Death, sitting quietly beside me, my own loud life-breath contrasting noisily in my ears.

Life made more textured and palpable with the weight of death gently leaning in.

The dakinis I met there were the kind who cut through ego, drama, opinion, and small-mindedness—the attachment-crushing, cloud-jumping, mother hawk kind. Their voices were those of a primal cry, something older than human language.

As an enveloping panic from a fear of heights reached for me, this summit became a great charnel ground in the sky, a land of alchemical transformation for the creation/destruction cycle of all things. I perceived the realness of sickness, old age, and death, as well as the presence of radical rebirth and renewal. And resting in the crux of this paradox was the mystery of this constantly liquid present moment and a sense of being soaked into infinity.

With tangible honesty, I was overcome by the absoluteness of decaying bodies and meat falling away from bones. I sunk into the universality of us all becoming the Earth's mulch, like fallen mother redwoods, blessed to be the fertile remnants for smaller trees to sprout from.

This was the truth of grainy, cremated ashes floating on wind currents, poured into sacred spaces, and sinking into oceans.

I am not sure how long I lasted, given my anxiety about the possibility of falling. What felt like an hour was probably ten minutes. This was a lesson in fierce discomfort. But it was also filled with a sacred knowledge that the mystery of our lives and the flowering of our life force, cannot be contained, crated, or held in the circuitry of the mind.

Sliding inch by inch on my butt down the rubble heap until I reached the main path, I kissed the ground, a bit shocked about why I had been so scared to begin with. Yes, I was damn high up, but there was something else. What was it that I touched up there?

Summiting was a literal and figurative edge-walking. Understanding the value of the entire expanse of experience, was to not participate in some kind of selective denial or rejection. I was being asked to widen myself past the fences of familiarity to take a chance on exploring the territory of uncomfortable possibility.

Buddhist teacher and activist Joan Halifax describes her surprise in learning that "even in their degraded forms, Edge States can teach and strengthen us, just as bone and muscle are strengthened when exposed to stress, or if broken or torn, can heal in the right circumstances and become stronger for having been injured."[5] According to Halifax, such states include altruism, empathy, integrity, respect, and engagement. She observes how freedom emerges from states of being where courage and fear meet. And it is exactly at these junctions that the dakini energies within us like to gather.

So be on the lookout for the Space Dancer in yourself. You do not need to attach her to a certain religious or spiritual path. Call on her essence, her spirit, her mysterious heart. She embodies freedom above all else. Be on the lookout for flesh and blood versions of the Space Dancer too, who might show up as a friend wise beyond her years or the kind of teacher that knows how to lovingly lean you into your limits.

Work with your inner Space Dancer (and all of the archetypal energies we are encountering in this chapter) with the intention of felt sense. A *felt sense* is a physical experience of body awareness that encompasses and communicates the quality of every sensorial detail. This is what it means to be embodied, to live and breathe more intentionally in your physical form.

Begin to work with how it feels to perceive through all of your senses versus just through your head. Make it all come *alive* within you.

Close your eyes now. The voice of the Space Dancer whispering in your ear is the revolutionary. But don't confuse her with a vigilante or an anarchist. She is sharp, clear, and purposeful. Strong. Focused. Confident. She may look like a stiff soldier, but she is really a peace activist cutting through all the extraneous distractions. Her voice echoes and calls to you as the sound of the wind howling down the mountains.

Setting yourself up with a quiet mind through a few minutes of meditation or breathing into your belly, take out your journal and begin to write on these questions.

- *The Space Dancer is like an untamed, unpredictable lightning bolt, flashing you with her force, waking you up. She asks you to contemplate what it would mean to leave the dry home of your comforts and go dance in the aliveness of your storm.*

- *As a follow-up question, think of some situation in your life where you would like to act but feel too afraid. Expanding yourself out wider to make space for the places you feel certain, or terrified, chaotic, or assured, free write on the question: "Where do fear and courage meet?"*

- *Reflect on any life experiences that remind you of how you became "stronger for being injured." Just like the knitting back of bones, free write on how these injuries wove a strength into your very tissues.*

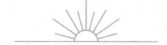

"I came to realize that the dakinis are the undomesticated female energies—spiritual and erotic, ecstatic and wise, playful and profound, fierce and peaceful—that are beyond the grasp of the conceptual mind. There is a place for our whole feminine being, in all its guises, to be present."[6]
—LAMA TSULTRIM ALLIONE

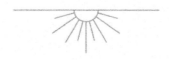

Call in the Inner Healer

There it is again. Pushing its delicate, pitcher-like petals towards the sun, presenting a patchwork of purple patterns across my yard and into the meadow edges. This small "weed," *Prunella vulgaris*, also known as *self-heal*, has a persistence and a strong will to spread, like so many other plant beings in the mint family. This plant teacher is well-named, for the force that we all contain to mend and heal is also amazingly tenacious.

You get a papercut. In a few days it's gone. You bash your shin on the bedpost. The bruise fades on its own. This is a phenomenon we all possess and rarely appreciate. Your body knows how to take care of itself. The speed and ease with which the body performs these miraculous repairs leaves these changes so often unnoticed.

Our bodies *want health*. And they are designed to ceaselessly return to a state of balance, if we choose to live in a way that supports and strengthens this innate power. Our bodies possess an inherent intelligence to self-diagnose and regenerate.

You break a bone, the most solid tissue of the body, and a straightforward fracture will resolve in a few months. Often those bone cells come together at the break site in such a miraculous and clever way that the fracture will no longer show up on an x-ray.

But how does our physical system, seemingly steeped in chaos and variability, always know how to come back to this place of balance?

This self-healing power within us is no different from the force that keeps the planet spinning or the drive of a plant to longingly lean itself towards the sun. It's the power behind a newborn baby humpback whale immediately searching for its mother's nipple to nurse after birth. Or the impulse of a salmon to swim upstream, against every odd and obstacle, to reach its original spawning grounds. The spark and will to *live*. This force penetrates and connects all things, from the tiniest single-celled organism to the entire universe.

The ancient Chinese called this force *qi*. Qi is the animating energy that drives all activity and change in the cosmos. In every culture and medical tradition before our current time, there has been an understanding that all living creatures contain vital energy. In many ways, the medicine of these ancient traditions couldn't be more futuristic or relevant for the times we live in.

Although our self-healing nature is always with us, it is not limitless. You cannot get four hours of sleep every night, drink Red Bull for breakfast, and smoke a couple of packs of cigarettes a day for years on end, and just figure your good old self-healer will take care of it. Many a rock star has tried this out already (and we know what results).

The gift of the archetype of the Inner Healer is about presence, choices, and deep listening. How conscious are you in the choices you make about your home or work environments, the people you surround yourself with or the kind of job that consumes your time?

This sense of presence and awareness concerns your physical body, too. Your body is constantly giving you hints and messages about how to best take care of yourself, but are you really paying attention? Do you hear your body's voice?

In my work as an acupuncturist, I constantly tend the temple grounds of the Inner Healer. I guide people in learning to listen to the whispers of this part of themselves, the part that knows what bedtime makes them feel most rested, the part that knows that a job is systematically killing them, or the part that knows why they are really sick. Sometimes this wisdom is subtle and hard to perceive and other times it is just painfully obvious. You get diarrhea every time you eat dairy? Well, I think you already know what you need to do.

Why do we not listen to our Inner Healers? I have wondered a lot about this over the years. Yes, we are inundated by our distracted minds, but this goes beyond not being in our bodies, not paying attention, not hearing. Why do we fight against what is best for us, even when we only hurt ourselves in the end?

Sometimes it is related to the "bad rebel" part of us, which has a self-disparaging bent. Other times we are triggered by experiences in childhood, and we are seeking control—not wanting to be told what to do. Kind of like an inner, unconscious foot stamping. Or we may just be plain pissed to have to limit our lives in some way. To have to limit our diets, limit our excessive doing, or limit our indulgences. This can be based on an inability to see the long-term view, to not perceive on a daily basis the way our choices may be slowly injuring us.

Perhaps we never received the education, training, or positive imprinting that would allow us to set up healthy habits or know how to take care of ourselves appropriately. Maybe we just don't think it's worth it—that we're not worth it.

It is just basic human nature that we orient by the here and now. Even though the Inner Healer tells us how to best take care of ourselves for our entire lives, we tune out this wisdom for what is momentarily sweeter, easier, or more comfortable. Often, we are trying to fill some endless hole within ourselves, that part of ourselves that is never quite satisfied, never quite full.

Resting deep within what is most settled and content in us, the voice of the Inner Healer rings with authenticity and awareness. Her tones link and sync up your gut, your heart, and your mind—all your avenues for inner knowing—so that they can work together. The intuition of the Inner Healer doesn't just know what we need for healing, she knows what we need to truly live well. She is unconcerned with lingering in imbalance and illness; she only knows the path to reorienting us in health.

She is a stubborn, unflinchingly honest guide. The voice of your Inner Healer will resonate with the truth no matter the source from which it comes, no matter how much you like it or not, and no matter what the consequences to your life might be. Like the outspoken voice of the Space Dancer, her inner truth cuts with a straightforward blade.

She lets us know where our emotional boundaries lie, such as when something feels unsafe or does not belong to us. She squirms when we are taking on other people's problems as our own. She itches when she perceives that our stories about ourselves are untrue or when she catches us going down rabbit holes of self-deprecation. She howls when we are engaging in unequal energy exchanges.

This is an especially important lesson for those who want to give over their power to or abdicate their responsibility of healing to others, doctors and other healthcare practitioners alike. Often, such people have given up the belief in their capacity to be well; they have forgotten that they too hold an essential role in caring for themselves.

What a gift she is. At her essence lies the capacity to become involved with and take responsibility for our individual healing journey. No variety of outer measures or restorative techniques can bring about genuine mending at any level unless we are quickened from within to seek the wholeness of life.

The Inner Healer is only as accurate as the depth of our presence and listening. In my professional practice, I have learned to work with the Inner Healer as an actual presence, a helping spirit that I can call upon and engage with on a daily basis.

INNER HEALER MEDITATION

Try this exercise as a way to connect deeper with your Inner Healer.

In a moment of quiet, steady yourself, grounding in your breath and feeling the solidness of whatever is below you, such as the floor, a bed, a chair, or the earth. Slow it all down.

Get into a space of connection and creativity, knowing that imagination is what your mind's energy rides on. From your own inner wisdom, with your eyes closed, call out to your Inner Healer. Ask her to come forward, revealing herself in form.

Let an image come into your mind and observe her every detail. Breathe in this meeting, noticing how you feel and how you interact with the energy. Make a gesture of connection in your mind, whether it be through an offering (giving of a small biodegradable gift, like flowers) or through touch. Just be watchful and available for a little bit. When the Inner Healer is ready to leave, take a moment to give thanks.

Then write down all of your observations. The age that your Inner Healer presents itself as reflects the maturity of your relationship together or how much energy in your life you have dedicated to this idea of self-healing. The health, or vibrance, of the Inner Healer also mirrors the well-being of the relationship. Maybe there is some repair work or apology that needs to be given because of past neglect.

This process is about making a joyful commitment to dedicate awareness to your self-love and self-care, the bedrock qualities that support feminine confidence. Nourish this relationship with the importance it deserves. You may feel the voice of the Inner Healer inside you as an intuitive fluttering, subtle and persistent, in your throat, chest, or belly.

Deepen your connection with your Inner Healer through practice, visualization, and journaling. Take out your journal right now and see what arises when your heart feels into these questions:

- *What gets in the way of you not hearing or not listening to your Inner Healer?*

- *What does your Inner Healer really have to say about the wheel of your life: your work, environments, hobbies, relationships, health, finances/resources, and mental/emotional landscape?*

- *What are some ways, ritualistic or otherwise, that you could connect with, honor, nurture, and hold gratitude for this great well of wisdom inside of you?*

"Living in touch with our inner guidance system involves feeling our way through life using all of ourselves: mind, body, emotions, and spirit. . . . We have to give our bodies credit for their innate wisdom. We also don't need to know exactly why something is happening in our bodies in order to respond to it. You don't need to know why your heart is racing or why you feel like crying. Understanding comes after you have allowed yourself to experience what you're feeling."[7]

—CHRISTIANE NORTHRUP

Call in Wild Gaia

Come put an ear to the ground. Make contact. Listen with *all* your senses. It comes from the mud. The dirt, soil, humus, bog, the land.

What lies beneath, buried in the rich, black butter? Something fertile and full. Deep beneath the worms and sleeping animals. Beneath the crystal caverns and dinosaur bones. This is the level at which we can no longer feel the impact of modern humans. There is a pulse, a heavy footstep, a drumbeat. These secrets will not be given easily, but there is a calling for us to uncover them, nevertheless. There is a dancing circle of elders, chanting, singing, interacting.

Calling to us.

This is not a journey to discover but one of *remembering*. This is to unabashedly know in our cells how deeply enmeshed we are in the continuance of life on this planet—to take our seats as luminous beings in an interconnected matrix. We are wild creatures still in our hearts, and if we listen really well, we can remember how to sing the song of nature.

We can learn the rain like the clouds know the sky.

We can call the names we hear on the river's currents.

We can feel and know the Earth within ourselves and ourselves within the Earth.

There is something very primal about interacting through the sense of touch, to feel the warm earth between your fingers, to befriend all the little organisms there. When I do this, I notice how it slows the pace of my life to the speed of the planet turning and the secret push of the grass upwards.

Planting and touching the land with my hands, is a work that reconnects me. Not just to the physical soil but to the power in the blood that pulses through the members of my female line. Guaranteed, even when any other conversation has run dry in my family, there is always more to share about the land, plants, gardens, or animals. Despite being such different humans, women from different generations with radically different ways of moving through the world, the thread that binds and weaves us together is our mutual love of growing things.

Many times, I have watched my mother's dirt-lined fingernails blissfully move about her tasks, nimbly snipping at an overzealous tomato start or tucking sunflower seeds deep into the little dirt pockets of their egg carton bed. Somehow her imprecise ease, her complete trust in all things to fight toward life has always turned true. Even the yellowest, driest, most miserable plant being would come to life for her, to sprout, to blossom, to burst for her.

My mother recently recounted to me how there is something about when her physical body gets into a certain position, back bent, legs crouched, and focused on her task, that she is transported to a certain feeling state with an ample peace. I guess you could equate it, as the closest thing, to a past-life vision—this sense of having touched the soil in this way, over and over and over again.

I also experience this portal of closeness. It's as if the flow and intimacy that planting, pulling, and digging provides is a therapy that I have relied on for a lot longer than this one short life.

In her beautifully written book *If Women Rose Rooted,* Sharon Blackie describes how women were the original gatekeepers and protectors of the land. She says: "It's no accident that the systemic suppression of the feminine has been accompanied down the centuries not only by the devaluation of all that is wild and instinctual in our own natures, but by the purposeful destruction of natural ecosystems."[8]

Western philosophy, over the last 2,000 years, has been feeding us the illusion of separation and supremacy. The lie goes something like this: humans are separate from nature. Not just separate, but also superior—*above it.* Reason and intellect are the unique skills of man and make men superior to everything else. The emotional and intuitive qualities of women placed them in this lesser-being category, on par with the beasts and critters.

The long-term effects of singularly clinging to an extremely distorted masculine orientation have played out in greedily taking more than our share, ruling with a plundering, dominating strong arm, in aggression and warfare and possession that have been pushing us past the brink.

The state of our current ecological emergency exposes a huge cultural falsehood that we still hold. This is the assumption that confidence rests in direct opposition to humility. This is to uphold a belief that strength only comes when we are wielding some hulking control and power over another. But the trouble with confidence that is untempered by humility is that it ends up as a stinking heap of unjustified arrogance. And somehow this myth of arrogance has been propagated, grown, and encouraged. We take and we take and we take, with an attitude of careless extraction instead of reciprocity—our bloated, hollow bellies never quite full.

This broken truth of separation and male authority could not be clearer in our modern lives. But even spanning back many years, D.H. Lawrence described it as "bleeding at the roots, because we are cut off from the earth and sun and stars, and love is a grinning mockery, because, poor blossom, we plucked it from its stem on the tree of Life and expected it to keep blooming in our civilized vase on the table."[9] Maybe it would just be easier if we kept our flowers plastic: no bleeding, no mess—so very civilized.

Our overzealous worship of domestication has even tried to turn our dirt clean. I look around neighborhoods at the bluish-green lawns, fertilized, trimmed, and edged, and I feel the depth of our spiritual barrenness. Leaf blowers batter the Earth, leaving it inert and stripped, contained and somehow more virtuous. Perfect rows of nonnative plants line up with no function, no food to provide, no way of interacting with the other plants around them—strangers in a strange land.

I see starvation, a sad hunger, for all the creatures, birds, and insects that are eking it out in these places, many populations now extinct or struggling to find food. I can also feel the strength of these resilient beings, making their way in these anemic, soulless ecosystems.

On an even larger scale, overgrazing and deforestation have led to immense amounts of soil erosion in the nineteenth and twentieth centuries. Permaculture expert Ben Falk describes how "topsoil is washing off the exposed heartland of America at a rate of about one billion dump-truck loads per year. Only a comet or large asteroid collision with Earth has ever destroyed so much biological capital so quickly."[10]

What does all of this sterility, this ecological exploitation, this containment of the wild within the living world, reflect about our expectations to tamp down the trembling heat of our own feral natures? How have we copied or even embodied these spirit-strangling restrictions within ourselves?

Because down below the surface layers, down in the black soil roiling with invisible skeins of microorganisms, down where only scientific listening devices can pick up the subtle vibrations of the oceans swishing and the humming of the globe turning, is where we find the essence of the dark feminine, the deep feminine, that buried feminine aspect of ourselves that cannot be controlled or pared back.

The wise feminine understands and accepts the irony in this truth: Growth begins in the dark. Because seeds are nourished by the moist cocoon of blackness, first moving their roots down before slowing drawing their sprout upwards. A forming child is fed in the shadowy penumbra of the womb, its black waters an imprint of boundless peace. Despite our conditioning to be scared of the dark and to be intimidated by the unknown depths within ourselves, the rich soil is the natural birthplace of feminine confidence.

The archetype of Wild Gaia wants you to find the confidence that rests here, at the very root of your root. She wants you to plant the seeds of your dreaming, your passions, your loves, deep into the teeming soil at the heart of you and see what will grow in its patient mystery.

Wild Gaia also wants us to make contact, wants us to know that beyond our all-important busyness lays the truth of the hollow loneliness in western culture. She encourages us to study and respect the wisdom of Indigenous lines of healing and insight throughout the globe, which have always believed in a net that connects every living thing, everywhere.

The shamanic teacher Sandra Ingerman uses this analogy: "We are like fingers of a hand that have dropped to the floor and who think they have a life of their own. For our health and for that of the planet, we must once again remember that we are part of a collective energy field, not separate from it."[11]

How can we begin to remind all those little floating fingers out there on their own to come to join their wizened hand? They are so much more powerful working as one.

Every breath we take, every swallow of water, everything we eat comes from the Earth. We travel through the Earth's atmosphere like whales through the ocean. We live *in* her body, not just *on* her body. We are made up of the very same elements: fire, earth, air, and water. We mimic and reflect her.

The mirror is being held higher now, as the current state of our ecological crisis is an ongoing reflection of our own psychological state. Our reticence to care for her is reflected in our inability to lovingly care for ourselves. We have stopped feeling nurtured by the Earth because we no longer belong to her. And if we no longer belong to her, than we no longer feel responsible in our relationship with her. Enmeshing ourselves within the web of the living world is to put a salve on all the places we have lived cut off, disembodied within ourselves.

For it is in connecting and returning to the other-than-human world that you are also returning to *yourself*.

I see you growing branches and roots now. Time to close your eyes and call in the archetypal energy of Wild Gaia, the essence of Mother Earth inside you. Find a quiet space in some sort of natural setting, even a city park or a balcony, and, in a state of openness and receptivity, ask to visit this part of yourself. Cultivate your longing to know her.

Through your "strong eye," your inner sight, set an intention of meeting with her. Let an image of her take form. What does she look like? How does she act? How does she move? Does she have any messages for you? Feel every detail and be open to what she wants to share with you. How can she best interact with and support your ongoing practices?

Once you have connected to the Wild Gaia archetype, take out your journal and explore these questions.

- *What are some examples of how your family and society have tried to control you, making you like a fertilized lawn—cut to perfection, doused in chemicals—squelching what is wild in you? What creature lives within you that wants to rebel against these constraints, or who knows what makes you feel most free?*

- *Poetry therapist Mary Reynolds Thompson, author of* Reclaiming the Wild Soul, *asks the very potent question: What if the desperate healing of "rewilding the Earth began with rewilding our souls?"[12] Reflect on the ways you have become estranged from the Earth, the great grief of this loss that we all share. It is so easy to feel crushed by the enormity of this communal task, this fragile homecoming to ourselves and to this planet. What if healing really does start within? What would this feel or look like for you?*

- *What does the paradigm of the natural world have to teach you about feeling into your intrinsic wholeness?*

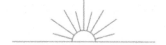

"By climbing up into this head and shutting out every voice but his own, 'Civilized Man' has gone deaf. He can't hear the wolf calling him brother—not Master, but brother. He can't hear the earth calling him child— not Father, but son. He hears only his words making up the world. . . . No use teaching women at all, they talk all the time, of course, but never say anything. This is the myth of Civilization, embodied in the monotheisms which assign soul to Man alone."[13]

—URSULA LEGUIN

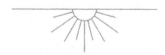

Call in the Artist-Visionary

Why do we call the Earth the Great Mother? Because she is the ultimate creator, always growing, the giver and sustainer of life. The Andean people use the term *Pachamama,* which literally translates as "World Mother." In their native culture, she is thought to be the quintessential fertility goddess, presiding over farming, the harvest, crops, and the uncontainable beauty of all living things.

We can instantly connect with the true importance of her power with the thought of emptiness ringing through our bellies. Nothing brings the seriousness of the harvest into full focus better than our own physical hunger. Without food, we have nothing. Cultures since the beginning of time share similar versions and stories of their local fertility goddesses. The Great Goddess is always the preeminent expression of creativity: nourishing breasts, full bellies sprouting, swelling, stretching, and giving life.

The life-giving, creative spark lives in all of us. Whether it be through cooking a gorgeous dinner, creating an adventurous bedtime story for your child, or doodling during a conference call, we all express creativity in some way in our lives. In fact, many of us are "closet creatives," unwilling to actually associate our biggest loves as some version of inner genius.

This was true for me. I caught the edges, the vague shadows of creativity occasionally in moments with my family, or in hidden, off-handed ways at work. But there was no connection made, no realization that I needed to give myself the allowance to let my creative juices flow forth. This archetypal energy was there all along, but I just couldn't *see it* within myself.

In a surprising shift, a light bulb of insight turned on when I was ready and I began to see all of the ways in which I was creative, much of the time. I was soaking in luscious pools of creativity; I just hadn't realized I was wet.

Then the question "Why not?" started to throb in my ears.

Why can't I dream myself differently than how I have thought of myself in the past?

Why, why, why not? Why can't I try on a different skin for a while?

So often we think of ourselves in a very static, one-dimensional way. Favorite ice cream flavor—chocolate. Favorite dish—pad thai. Hair only looks good—shoulder length. Can only live—in the desert. We compartmentalize the holy life out of ourselves, all the way down to what we think we are good at and what is worth doing.

There is a guest room in my mother's house that is overflowing with stacks of albums, peeling collages, and chipped picture frames memorializing the many stages of her children. And I don't know if it feels more like a shrine or a crypt—maybe both. When I enter this room, I am overwhelmed by all of the various versions of myself, all of the many times I have stripped my skin and birthed myself anew. I am so grateful that I can squeeze out of all of the dried skins of who I think I am, all of the many places in my mind that I am still trapped in the copper frames of pictures taken when I was six, or eleven, or twenty-five. The words of essayist Joan Didion remind me, "I have already lost touch with a couple of people I used to be."[14]

Stepping into the land of the Artist-Visionary, she tells me to please, please, please continue to dream myself fresh. She asks me to create a pile of crusty sheddings, long, lingering doubts, and qualities I assumed I would have forever. Just lay it all down, all those beliefs that are like grungy clothes that no longer fit.

The Artist-Visionary tells us to let curiosity be our torch. She reminds us that we can find everything around us interesting if we choose to see it that way—because creativity invites us to travel beyond our ordinary limits of language and experience. It asks us to check our egos at the door. If we dare, it allows us to cross a bridge into a place of magic and mystery that we didn't know existed. It is this creativity that ultimately connects us to the shiny essence of what makes us gorgeous, flawed human beings.

For it does not live in the completion, in the finished portrait or the filled-up journal. It is in the making, the ever-unfolding, ongoing exploration of joy. Art does not want us to be comfortable or bored or static. It wants us to be so awake that we are able to actually catch every little firefly of insight that wanders within view.

This is because creativity encourages us to live life *amplified*. I feel creativity to be like a sprite, an essence, an energy, a flow, instead of a solid process. In the way that it moves, stirs, and ignites us, it is always transforming potential into manifestation. It is not some limited resource to be put on a high shelf far from reach, but something to be swayed with, immersed in all of the time.

If you only use your creativity in one area of your life, this energy can become tightly partitioned. But the more your creative essence flows through all areas of your life, the more it acts as a unifying force that weaves together the complete experience of your life's potential. Like water ungoverned, it has this way of moving through all our tributaries, the veins of skinny creeks, generous tributaries, and widely etched rivers. It is this flow, across the entirety of your life, that sustains and continually fuels you up.

Psychoanalyst Clarissa Pinkola Estés continues with this theme of creative waters: "Creating one thing at a certain point in the river feeds those who come to the river, feeds creatures far downstream, yet others in the deep. Creativity is not a solitary movement. That is its power. Whatever is touched by it, whoever hears it, sees it, senses it, knows it, is fed."[15] It is ripples and ripples of rainwater on a still lake, circles reverberating endlessly.

So, take a moment now to ask yourself: What are the biggest hurdles that stand in the way of connecting with your most creative life? Most often what separates a mundane existence from one of color and curiosity is a willingness to (once again) listen to our fear. Our fear of falling apart, or making a mess, or hanging out in chaos, or being a fool. As Elizabeth Gilbert says in her book *Big Magic:* "We all know that fear is a desolate boneyard where our dreams go to desiccate in the hot sun."[16]

What creative dreams do you have that are wasting away in that boneyard right now? In order to enter the sacred ground of the Artist-Visionary, you must call all your little (or gigantic) fears out into the open so that they can be fully seen and acknowledged.

Maybe you think someone else will always do it better. That you have nothing original to share. This is the trap of dirty comparison.

Maybe you think art is for kids and you will feel silly or exposed in some way. This is ego standing in the way of freedom.

Maybe you feel like you just don't have time or that it is unproductive, like creativity is some form of egotism.

Or maybe you think you don't deserve it. Perhaps you have an old belief that you are not worthy of experiencing pleasure and play.

Come on, get it all out into the open. The confidence inherent in the Artist-Visionary is based in witnessing these fears and in turn, upholding the sustaining, life-giving power that creativity brings. Every time we actually identify and expose our fears to the light of day, we take away their heaviness, we shrink them. We hold fear by its hand, look it in the eyes and more fully acknowledge how it is keeping us captive. And we acknowledge how we may have been using up creative energy by applying our *old* stories to a *new* situation or potential.

How can the creative act be used to feed the deepest desires of your soul? It is vital to ask this question because, as Julia Cameron describes in *The Artist's Way*: "Our creative dreams and yearnings come from a divine source. As we move toward our dreams, we move toward our divinity."[17] Expressing our creativity is to recognize that we hold a sacred place in the cycle and order of life; that we ourselves are creations, which then, in turn, flourish and create some more.

How can you use this natural resource to process your unacknowledged, unconscious life's material, composting it into something beautifully revealing, maybe even heart-openingly healing? Living a creative life allows us to better adapt to sudden changes or unexpected breakdown. It acts as an underground aquifer of resourcefulness and improvisation so that maybe we can get just a little more fluid with all of life's experiences.

Her voice, like some ethereal expression of water, the Artist-Visionary wants to connect with you now. Taking out your journal, what truths rise to the surface when you write on these questions:

- *How can you take play more seriously (wink, wink)? With gentle, deliberate effort, how can you nourish your artistic inner child, to be willing to know beauty, humor, and joy to be just as important as hard work?*

- *What would it take to forge a lasting creative awakening in your life? What blocks are standing in your way right now?*

- *How might the energy of water help you better understand and know more creativity in your life, which you can then pass along and share with others?*

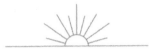

"Creativity isn't just about knitting scarves or going on painting courses; it isn't about creating great works of art or writing bestselling books. Creativity is an authentic approach to life: an openness, a spontaneity; a determination to nurture rather than destroy."[18]

—SHARON BLACKIE

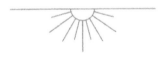

The Confidence of the Four Sentries

Walking the wilds of yourself, the essence of the four archetypal energies offers you reminders of your inner resources, especially in those slippery moments of doubt, darkness, or forgetting. Familiarize yourself with each one, calling on them individually as your life asks.

The confidence of the Space Dancer reminds you to feel your uncertainty (and the way it wants to plead, cling, and continually pin you in place), bringing you to the intersection of courage and fear. You may find it particularly useful to connect with her in times of sudden or substantial change in your life, any forms of edge walking, transition, or reinvention.

The confidence of the Inner Healer reminds you to trust your inner-knowing; she echoes to you that you are wiser than you realize. You may reach out to her when you are wanting to strengthen your intuition, self-care, sense of embodiment, or to enhance your connection to your overall health and well-being.

The confidence of Wild Gaia reminds you to connect in with your older, wilder creature self. You may call on her when you feel lost or overwhelmed by the world; she reconnects you to the Earth, to your own naturalness, wonder, and desire. She encourages you to tune in to the greater rhythms, your core values, and to the expansiveness of your soul.

The confidence of the Artist-Visionary reminds you to hold your creativity and curiosity as sacred and essential to a well-lived life. You may find her when you have been working too hard, teetering on burn-out, lost in the pushing, or stuck in self-doubt. She helps to instill a fluidity to your life, opening a forgotten flow of ease, joy, and pleasure.

They are sovereign natives, fully inhabiting their space as they teach you about friction and the bravery it takes to sometimes step off the well-worn path of cultural assumptions, reinventing your understanding of what it means to be a woman. Their voices are valid, bold, and unique in their own right, manifesting the many different expressions of the fierce feminine.

May the sound of their wisdom/your wisdom keep echoing in your ears as we plunge further into our journey together, finding the impassioned voice of the body.

CHAPTER FOUR

Voice of the Body

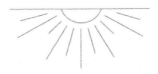

"Before you can hear, much less follow, the voice of your soul, you have to win back your body. You have to go on a pilgrimage beneath the skin."[1]
—MEGGAN WATTERSON

What gorgeous, meaty animals we are. These precious skins that breathe and protect, these sinews that ache to stretch, these senses that constantly teach us the language of delight. Swerve, curve, grow, bend, bow—our physical bodies rival any other miracle found in nature. The revelation of their magic is up there with frost flowers on winter lakes, the smoke that thunders off waterfalls, and the bubble, pop, and fizz of cerulean blue ice. The inner workings of our mitochondria and electric hearts, and the symphonies of our hormones are just as mysterious as dark matter matrices, the deepest marine trenches, and the blooming of polar fringe flowers.

Home

We get so few opportunities to truly reflect on and connect with this blessing of a body. Layers of flesh, gristle, tendon, organ, blood, bone—so vital, so assumed, so loved, so hated.

Our bodies are arguably the most important gifts we will ever be given. And yet it is strange to realize that while we are completely obsessed with our bodies, we remain simultaneously largely disconnected from them. As women, we are preoccupied with dressing them up, shaping them down, plucking, primping, and painting them into submission. But despite all of the surface-level attention, they remain out of touch, a bit alien to us.

This relationship of foreignness is natural in the beginning, excusably appropriate. Shafts of light, vague shapes, and brief swishes of motion are the only things we see when we first come into this life. Like so many other creatures that are born looking pitiful, squinty, and undeveloped, humans emerge into a nondescript world. When our eyes start to focus more clearly, however, we immediately begin to interact, to reach out. We start to stretch our hands toward faces, shiny mobiles, and of course, our own plump toes.

This toe-grasping is our first real interaction with our own tender bodies. But to a young baby, those readily available, fleshly feet seem like just another toy, a fun thing to grab.

Something entirely separate.

The difficulty remains that for many of us we carry on through the rest of our lives with this very same perspective of the body as something detached from ourselves. We come to see it as a smooth pumping machine with compartmentalized pieces. A tissue-covered engine made to do our bidding. We don't know how to listen to what our bodies really need or want.

Even as adults, there exists a persistent, foggy conundrum: We don't really know how to inhabit ourselves well.

The discordance we maintain with our bodies seems to be becoming ever more extreme; our modern lifestyle is turning us into a bunch of large craniums walking around on stick legs. Days speed by under the leadership of our filled-to-the-brim heads, which end up overwhelmed and overworked like massive, smoking turbines. We are addicted to the opium glow of our screened devices, to the seduction of their stimulation and movement. A cultural terror has spread among us in our extreme avoidance of being still.

Even the most basic of body functions—eating, drinking, peeing, pooping, resting, deep breathing, and sleeping—can be forgotten in this blur. How can we feel truly *incarnated,* living more fully in the flesh? How do we learn to go into ourselves, to know *intimacy* (into-me-see) with the deepest depths of our being?

In order to explore these questions more fully, we must be willing to make the sensitive, but essential shift in our thinking from *having* a body to *being* body. We must stop treating our form as a thing—a warm lump of sorts—and come to know ourselves as enmeshed and integrated *as* our bodies.

I deeply resonate with the body wisdom of Zen writer Susan Moon and I refer to her words often: "I don't want to *have* a body anymore. I want to be it. I don't want to carry it around. I don't want to look out through it as if though chinks in a wall. I don't want it to be my pimp, to send it out looking for people to bring home to love me. . . . I don't want to treat it like an enemy soldier when it causes me pain and fight back with chemical warfare. I don't want to lie in bed, trembling and alone *beside* it, as if beside a sullen lover who refuses to be cheered. I'm tired of having a body. I just want to be my body."[2]

She poetically captures the subtle beliefs we carry of body as object, property, luggage, even adversary. Oh, how we love to keep body as foe. I feel in her words the deep exhaustion at the heart of maintaining this illusion. It is so very tiring to separate ourselves this way. Transcending a sense of alienation, your body can be more than a flesh house— it can be the more fully embodied you.

The truth is that our understanding of body is messy and nuanced: body can be identity, it can be gender, it can be pain, it can be ecstasy, it can be a vehicle of liberation, it can be aging and death. For all of these reasons, it makes sense to me that some people on a spiritual path may be tempted to skip over the body entirely. They share a belief that if we were really illuminated, we should be able to just slide past all the complicated trappings of having a physical form and jump straight into knowing each other as light beings. They might wonder, *Can't we just leave the body behind?*

For women (or any other humans who have experienced racism or discrimination based on their outward form), the body cannot be ignored, cannot be conveniently overlooked. Because it is in this bypassing of the body that we also gloss over the very real suffering that these tender bodies have endured. We also entirely miss the possibility of allowing our bodies to act as their own crucial portal of awareness. So often we fail to see the way our small, individual bodies connect us to the bigger body of all of life and the universe.

Instead of seeking to separate or elevate ourselves above our bodies, let us use them as much-needed opportunities of spiritual exploration. Continued consideration of race, sexuality, and gender bring us closer to our essence, not further isolated from it. Author and Zen Buddhist teacher Zenju Earthlyn Manuel describes: "If we do not anchor our inquiry into life within the undeniable, physical reality in which we live, spiritual awakening will remain far too abstract."[3] I feel her words putting rocks in the pockets of our spiritual lives, bringing us back down to the Earth.

The closest thing that we may get to the ultimate truth rests here, in each embodied moment. Connecting with and fully inhabiting our bodies presents us with a direct opportunity to know our humanness.

And it is in the sometimes tedious, sometimes rapturous quality of earthly moments that we may come into direct relationship with our own previously unappreciated sanctity. Yes, even in this moment of struggle, or dreaming, or frustration, or disintegration, or doubting, or plotting, or loving, we can accept ourselves with the warm arms of a benevolent confessional.

In this way, true embodiment relies on a certain confidence and courage to show up in experiencing our world exactly as it is. This is to slow, observe, and listen to precisely what is arising for us in that moment, without a predetermined agenda. Inhabiting our bodies more mindfully grows our capacity to stay with what we are experiencing, which in turn allows us to befriend our physical form. The fluid interdependence of mind and body is like a mobius strip. Over time a deepening occurs in this circular relationship, a reinforced intermingling of body awareness, confidence, and self-trust.

What would it feel like to fully arrive in our bodies despite everything we may be feeling: our restlessness or dissatisfaction, our learned shame patterns, our society telling us that we are the wrong size, shape, color, or gender? Oh, and let's not forget the incessant, pernicious effects of sexual objectification. In many ways, the influence of the patriarchy may weigh hardest on us here, in the realm of the flesh. The 1,000-pound chain of our cultural programming wants to desperately wrap itself around our bending arms, our wandering legs. It longs to snarl up our movements and embed in our skin.

Freedom means no longer deferring our sense of orientation to these iron manacles. But we will better know where we are going by first understanding where we have been.

What are the ways that we still unconsciously apologize through our body language or posture? What are the shields that our bodies have learned to hold up in attempts to block microaggressions or sexual objectification? What have we been burying in our bodies over time, slowly shoveling, tucking away trauma and self-hurt into our earth? We can use these body "writings" to better understand where confidence lives in our physicality and identify what stands in the way of us knowing it.

This act of listening to the voice of the body, or taking a "pilgrimage beneath the skin," as feminist theologian Meggan Watterson describes it, is a practice as vital as any other spiritual habit we hold.[4] When we lean in closer, we might realize that the body always has a point of view. It just articulates its opinions in ways that we may not always hear or understand. Learning how to tune in to our own body as infinitely wise and complex—an entire galaxy of sacredness— is an essential part of awakening feminine confidence.

The Secret Life of the Body

Truly embodying ourselves requires an acknowledgement of the two-fisted paradox that, on the one hand, our bodies mean so much, and on the other hand, they mean so little. We must acknowledge that these cherished, impermanent constructions of clay are ever-morphing, -changing, -flaking, and -decaying.

Zen Buddhist teacher Jan Chozen Bays describes how "being born, clay is formed. Living clay bodies chip and gradually or suddenly! break down. Dying, they disintegrate into clay particles again, are gathered, kneaded, and made into new bodies. In the potter's studio are millions of vessel-bodies, continuously being formed, functioning according to their purpose, breaking down, being remade as something new. Nothing enters and nothing leaves."[5]

Let us hold a certain reverence for these majestic, maturing clay bodies of ours. This clay is of the Earth, and we are a part of its all-powerful recycling system. It is fruitless to resist. There is holiness in knowing how our bodies break down, in knowing that we are inevitably being pulled by some tremendous cyclical force—the undertow of life and death.

What a dear body endures, what it holds in all of the places that have turned more like stone than pulsing tissue—a lifetime of emotion held in our flesh—is like a mighty castle of accumulation. The body tells us much about how we have lived and what we have returned to again and again. The body reveals where we have placed our attention. What our time and energy has been devoted to. The kind of past we have lived. If we have prayed on our hands and knees. That which we have taken a shovel to and buried alive within us. That which has been hushed.

I love the land of soft flesh. After so many years of greeting different bodies as an acupuncturist, it is a special kind of comfort for me to swim within the waves of fascia with my fingers, curiously exploring what is held there. There is familiarity found within this compassionate sliding over cautious threads to expose knotted, sticky, knobbed, gritty, twisted, gummy holdings in the tissues. I am fascinated by the mystery of why tears, ticklishness, laughter, or squirming appear whenever we give attention to these skin-covered pockets of unconscious retention, these receptacles of feeling. The body seems to take a great sigh of relief when we bring acknowledgment to these forlorn island parts of ourselves, the muscles brightening with physical touch and care.

Sometimes I run a careful finger over my own bumps and bruises, trace the thresholds of my broken bones, pay tribute to my stretch-mark palaces, and contemplate my many scars. The lines of these patiently stoic markings feel to my touch like graves dug into my skin's surface long ago. This reflective gazing is done to witness the miracle of my body's cemeteries, which are woven over by scarred lines that rest like rows of fading pink flowers. I feel how the imperfect nature of these blemishes mark me as ever more living and whole—not less.

I imagine my curves of fat and tendon needing to be identified by a coroner, who will know me by the slender crepe ribbons of scar tissue on my knees and the half-moon of healed skin on the pad of my left middle finger. Also, by the very large mole I loathe on the small of my back. And the many covered-over holes along my left ear. These are the quiet healings of a rebellious teendom, when piercing holes in myself was my way of venting the raging lava of feeling that wanted to erupt from inside of me.

The body of a woman has so much to tell when it's invited into a conversation.

Perhaps the body of a woman speaks through its shape and line, like the simplicity of a pointer finger slightly bent, curved by the pressure of her repetitive grip upon her pen.

Or there is something expressed in her overly developed calves, legs desperately searching for ground and stability in a changeable world.

There are unsaid words in the shapeless and yielding skin of her breasts that long ago surrendered to the impertinence of a nursing child.

Her feet confess of being tortured prisoners in shoes too tight, too pointy, too sexily fashionable, now knobby and deformed from their years of tenure.

The noiseless expression of her upper back is curved with the suffering, the weighted bricks of extreme competence and incessant care-giving.

The skin of her hands has become worn and speckled like rotting fruit from a lifetime of washing, weeding, kneading, sewing, rubbing, scrubbing, chopping, and soaking out in the sun.

Ecofeminist Susan Griffin writes of a woman and how "her body is a fortress, her body is an old warrior . . . her body living its secret life, her body sheltering wounds, her body sequestering scars, her body a body of rage, her body a furnace, an incandescence, her body the exquisite fire, her body refusing, her body endlessly perceiving…"[6]

The female body is not just any body. It is a radiant fortress of life. An astonishing, fragile, ferocious temple of holy complexity.

In a way, our forms never lie. They do not lie about all they contain, the many strips of sediment—toxins, tensions, aches, pains, emotions, and all sorts of other experiences, especially traumas—lined up in ancient layers of basalt, granite, obsidian, and sandstone. There is so much that lies quietly underground in the secret life of a woman.

Sitting with nature, I sense all of the many intersections between the Earth and the female form. I see the bodies of women lying along the land's edge, curved and rolling mountain ranges in all shades of ruddy ocher and burnt umber. Lines highlighted from the falling, fading sun creating sepia grooves along the arc of hips, the bend of shoulders.

I watch how the sunset dresses these mountains in sensual color, rose blush on breast peaks, cinnamon brushed on gangly knees and elbows, scarlet and vermillion running through rivulets of rebellious, rocky hair. It feels endless, the unfolding contours, the flexing, twisting, arching movement of the Earth, so similar to the soft curves of a woman's body.

Breathe in a sense of gratitude for the wonder of your own body, ever miraculous, ever sophisticated, its contours mirrored in the tones and terrain of the Earth. For this moment, know your body to be a thing of sacred beauty, a goddamn masterpiece worthy of reverence and celebration.

More than any other archetype, it is the Inner Healer that shows up again and again in these body-confidence explorations. Calling on the Inner Healer as your guide right now, take out your journal and see what insights arise in response to these reflections and questions:

- *Consider the strength and resiliency of your body, in all that it contains and has experienced. Let a great wave of thanks wash over you for everything*

your body is. Unleash a river of gratitude for all of the miracles it performs
each and every day. Laying down the weights of any and all self-deprecation,
free write about your body as a creature of marvel.

- *What are the receptacle areas of your body, holding zones where you place*
  your tension and emotion? If your body could speak clearly to you instead of
  just shutting down when it is overwhelmed with feeling or pain, what would
  it tell you? And what might you answer in response?

- *Working with a sense of "being" a body versus just "having" a body, how*
  could incorporating more embodiment practices, such as yoga, martial arts,
  meditation, or breathing exercises, allow you to feel more connected with your
  body as home?

The Gristle of the Earlobe

One of the largest blocks that we women have against believing that
we are worth caring for well is our lineage of shame. Shame is like a
vandal that we have welcomed into the home of our bodies for years.
Every night we leave the light on and the door open for shame to
enter, its visitations set by the chiming of a hallway clock. The visits of
shame seem as normal as those of a distant relative or a family friend—
so much so that it is may later be introduced to our daughters, shaking
their hands as well.

But the truth is that shame does not inherently belong to us; we
were not born to question our value or our physical form. A pudgy
toddler has absolutely zero ambivalence about the genius of her arms
and legs, which are always available for gorgeous movement. She
doesn't realize it yet, but she loves this thing called body.

A toddler has not yet been crushed by the weight of the print,
online, and broadcast media's massive system of humiliation. She has
not yet witnessed millions of flashing images on television, posters,
computer screens, music videos, and magazines, geared up to convince

her of how she must/should appear. She does not yet know the bitter venom of comparison.

Shame takes its sweet time to infiltrate our minds. But what about the influences even closer to us, in the vulnerable cloisters of our childhood home?

What has your family taught you about the look of a woman in her naturalness, in both the blooming of youth and as changelings of decay? As Maya Angelou once said, "I believe that one can never leave home. I believe that one carries the shadows, the dreams, the fears, and dragons of home under one's skin, at the extreme corners of one's eyes, and possibly in the gristle of the earlobe."[7] How do these subtle influences of your past home (your family/your relations) still control how you feel in your current home of a body?

What have our mothers taught us about the divinity (or sacrilege) of our flesh?

In your own life, who were your role models for this? Who taught you about the sensuality and shiver of your nakedness? Has your mother ever shown her naked body to you? Has she ever felt steady enough, in the pit of her own marrow, to flaunt herself with everything included? Has she ever shaken the skin of her own vulnerability in front of you just to let you know she is unafraid?

My mother is not a nudist by any means, but even as a teenager I admired her openness in changing clothes in front of me, to let the skin of her five births show. There was a freedom she passed to me this way, an invisible gift. As a child, I would tenderly inspect her lines, her body so strong and full and foreign to me. Strange hair growing in strange places. The marks of time written along her muscles felt curious and formidable to my eyes. Her horsewoman's hands exuding their broad life force, their enduring skin loved like rubbed velvet.

My own daughter inspects me this way now. I have seen her watching. Nothing I do is lost under her steely, eagle-eyed gaze. I know what she is thinking because I had those same thoughts at her age. A grown woman's body seems so outlandish, so immense, so rugged to a child. It teems with an unfamiliar intensity, an inner power that seems to gather in strength with the weathering of life.

I walk my nakedness in front of her, and I offer her this present, this effigy of self-love. This is how I teach her to let her own skin always be the shape and size to fit her just right. To feel utterly comfortable with what she finds there. To disrobe from all the cultural prisons, to strip herself clean, and to witness what remains: her own inherent, bountiful completeness.

My form also teaches her about the life-cycle of a body, about how the years move along the skin. That even she, a peony bloom with a radiance so piercing and fresh right now, will come to know the ever-ripening passage of time.

Flowers present us with such an achingly honest expression of aging. There is no flower that is more dramatic and elegant in its transformation process throughout its lifespan than the coral bark peony. Starting off a tiny bud, bright magenta, petals folded in so tenaciously, she then begins to unfold her feathered layers, becoming more and more glorious with each fractal of pink luster she unfurls. To start so small, it can only be a miracle to swell and puff into such an expression of outrageousness.

But there is a turning point when the energy shifts, and from coral, her blush begins to fade. Every day, the peony's petals turn a new shade of peach as her color and life force slowly float away. When all her petals are on the table, pale white and silky, I find what remains to be mere plant bones and dust. The essence of her flower wisdom now blown back to the Earth.

Similar to the coral bark peony, women spend a short time in the crisp green of their youth and a long time in the magnificent ebbing of aging. A young girl stops growing in height a couple of years after her menses begin and the final circuitry of her brain is complete somewhere in her mid-twenties. She proceeds to spend many, many more decades in the slow ripening of the dying process. We spend the vast majority of our lives in this elegant, natural maturation, and yet our boxing gloves are out for most of that time, always fighting, wrestling, denying the truth of this unfolding.

The cycles of a woman's life represent just another opportunity to engage confidently with her embodiment. Each phase holds its own beauty, its own challenge, and its own learning. Ancient Celtic traditions have a particularly beautiful way of understanding these life stages: the young maiden was seen as the flower, the mother (of the creative years) was the fruit, and the elder woman, the holder of the seeds. Instead of thinking of these seeds as some dried up, brittle things, we can know these seeds to hold the knowledge and the potential for everything else.

Why do we perceive the aging and changing process within the living world as natural and yet fail to include ourselves in this view? Sitting among a sacred grove of Oregon white oaks, this thought picked away at me. Nestled among the drying piles of acorns and fallen leaves, I looked up to find massive, entangled limbs graciously shading me.

In the 1800s these trees lived in great savannahs throughout the Willamette Valley of Oregon, acting as an important part of the local ecosystem and providing an abundance of food to the Kalapuya Indigenous people. But over time about 99 percent of these groves have been overtaken with conifers, farms, and other types of development.[8]

Hiking more deeply into this grove, I came across the great-grandmother of their community, a 400-year-old heritage white oak. I was stunned to contemplate all she had witnessed. I did not think to criticize her outer appearance, gnarled limbs, knobby bulges, and strange trunk growth. It never even crossed my mind. Instead there was a torrent of awe in my head: to think of all of the fires she has lived through, the draughts she has endured, diseases she has healed from, and the loneliness she must have known in the loss of other trees around her. Her twisted arms raised towards the sky, she seemed to move with invisible currents in an expression of absolute creativity and flow.

Using the Wild Gaia archetype as your guide, now is the time to rewrite your ideas about the inherent naturalness of your body. Taking out your journal and connecting with your truth and intuition:

- *What would it feel like to be in your toddler body again? What does the young child in you have to tell you about a feeling of ease in your flesh?*

- *What teachings from your family line still live in you unconsciously, even in the "gristle of your earlobes?" You were not born with any predetermined beliefs about your body but you may have made them your own over time.*

- *Thinking back to the example of the coral bark peony, imagine if your body could live through the life cycle of a flower. What flower would you be and how might this change your view and acceptance of aging and decay?*

Shields

For so many women just getting to the point of simple self-acceptance can feel like a huge accomplishment. And it is. But is there more waiting for us? Can we know more than just acquiescence, which seems to have an unspoken tone of just barely tolerating ourselves? Because banishing body shame requires more than just plain self-acceptance or some watered-down version of passive resignation. We may think we are outsmarting our negative body self-talk by accepting what we have been given. But have we? Isn't this some kind of tolerating, a certain settling, another form of just getting by? And, oh my, have we just gotten by.

We've gotten by with potato chip meals, shitty bosses, and caustic partners. Gotten by with inhumane work hours and lewd, inappropriate comments and being forced to worship a male-version of God. There are so many, many ways we have settled, stuffed it down, or sucked it up. There have been so many times that we have closed something within ourselves in order to survive.

In her book *The Body Is Not an Apology,* spoken-word artist and social justice activist Sonya Renee Taylor describes how there is more available to us than just plain self-acceptance. She promises, "There is a richer, thicker, cozier blanket to carry through the world. There is a realm infinitely more mind-blowing. It's called radical self-love."[9]

Body shame is one of the most common ways that we turn the body into an "other." Embarrassment about our own forms creates a certain mutiny from the body. Sometimes, it is easier for us to banish or reject ourselves entirely than to do the painful work of self-love. It is a rebellious act to love ourselves despite a lifetime of training otherwise.

In her book, Taylor provides *unapologetic inquiries,* methods of questioning employed in order to begin the process of body shame dismantlement. When did we learn to hate our bodies? How have we allowed images from the media around us to guide and influence what we take as normal? How do we keep its commerce alive through our own "buying to be enough"? We buy makeup to cover up the "sins" of our faces, constraining garments to hide the way our "ugly" flesh wants to express itself, and shoes to make out asses sway "seductively" when we walk unsteadily through the world on them.

She offers tools for how we need to "dump the junk" of the commercial mass-media system and the toxic messaging it spews. Let us also catch our own perpetual bad mouthing of other women and our destructive self-talk to make space for new stories full of mercy and inspiration.

To start a new relationship with the body, we must first identify how we continue to apologize *through* our bodies. How we hide, excuse, or repent for our femaleness. The ways in which we cross, shield, cover ourselves. The false smiles we offer, the rigid jaws, hunched shoulders, and stiff muscles we front with, disguising all of the places we feel insecure, nervous, or unsure.

Holding up mirrors of honest inquiry, we can begin to notice the apologies in how our bodies speak. In the subtlest of details, our body language reveals, as body language expert Tonya Reiman says, the "differences between what a person says and what a person truly believes."[10] It takes awareness and attention to catch the edge of strain in your smile or the clenching in your right toe. There are so many ways that we women protect or wall ourselves off or get small through our physical expression.

I think of these conscious or unconscious body barricades as *shields*. Sometimes we set up these shields through our body language; other times, it is through wearing thick layers of makeup or building a layer of extra fat around our middle. A wall of excess flesh can be its own crafty, unconscious defense mechanism. But so too can a wall of pointy collar bones.

Even distractions in the form of excessive screen time can be its own form of shielding, allowing us to dissociate, to escape our bodies and what we are really feeling. These types of behavioral shields may feel comfortable at the moment, but they hide our tense undercurrents, and they reinforce a sense of distrust that radiates out into everything in our lives.

Let me make it very clear that there are many intelligent reasons why women have developed strategies to protect themselves emotionally and wall themselves off through their use of body language or other actions. We can, for example, be ogled, catcalled, felt up, or have our personal space invaded as we are just walking down the street. We know that at any moment our shields may have to go up. Having an arsenal at our disposal makes rational sense.

Even the way men and women look at each other can be different. According to Reiman, "Men tend to use hunt-vision, most pronounced in the up-and-down glance known as the once-over. In contrast, due to different brain wiring, women can more covertly take in a guy's entire body in one quick glance."[11] Women prefer subtlety, finesse, tact.

There is a stomach-lurching sensation that occurs when you realize that you are being made sexual prey. What do women sometimes do as a natural reflex? They cross their arms. They cross their legs. They cross their ankles. They find ways to shelter their bodies physically.

Women are deliberately taught to shroud themselves. This is to make sure our dangerous, unruly crotches are contained and impenetrable, our clandestine curves well-managed. But in any conscious or unconscious crossing of limbs or shying away from potential contact, we are always held just a little off balance, hips twisted, pelvis shifted, feet unevenly touching the floor.

Other anxious and defensive behaviors we may employ include turning, fidgeting, touching, tapping, swaying, picking, and shiftiness. Restlessness. These are the many ways that the female body says no. This body language could be saying, "No, I don't trust you," "No, I don't agree with you," or "No, back off because something you are doing is making me feel uncomfortable." Like a little barometer, these signals you're emitting could be like an early warning system letting you and everybody around you know how you really feel.

You may be like a wolf giving its warning growl.

When you sit with both feet on the ground, feeling the steadiness of the ground under you, it is actually a much safer and stronger way to be. The energy through your spine and head is able to run unblocked and uninhibited in this posture. And it reads more confidently to observers too. You are giving the person in front of you signals that you are awake, aware, and listening—that you are in your power.

The practice of embodiment helps us hear the unspoken words of our bodies. Over the course of the next few days, take some time to observe your body language, especially when you are with people you don't know or don't trust. Write down your observations in your journal. The intuitive nudging of the Inner Healer is with you again. Here are a few other suggestions:

- *Pay close attention to exactly what you do in your body when you feel uncomfortable, what kinds of crossing or shielding do you set up?*

- *When you observe your body, watch for any ways in which you might unconsciously apologize: a slight submissive forward folding through your chest or a tension in your jaw from smiling too hard. Imagine what your body would look like without this constant subtle armoring.*

Where Confidence Lives

For the sake of simplicity, we are now going to turn our exploration of feminine confidence toward four particular body areas: the pelvis, the backbone, the chest, and the eyes. There are so many places that confidence lives in the body; these areas were chosen for emphasis and ease.

Entire books have been written on analyzing and understanding these places in the body through both the lens of body-language interpretation and traditional systems of energy medicine. Mine will not be a complete or exhaustive inquiry of either of these types. Instead, I am looking to mark thresholds, to leave you cairns in clear places showing you where you could further focus your attention. I want you to move energy through these areas, knowing them to be open and vibrant.

It is our guardedness as women that ultimately shuts down our life force, leading us to feel like half-alive versions of ourselves. It is exhausting, even on an unconscious level, to always hold up our shields. We have excellent training in confining ourselves within our subtle straightjackets. We could be awarded doctorates in self-restraint.

It is damn near impossible to feel fully confident and at ease when we are chronically shut down and on-guard. In order to reclaim our power, we must bring ourselves fully back to life. We must better perceive what in us feels alive and what feels dead. We must connect with the unabashed freedom of our animal selves. The dialect of nature never speaks in tones of body shame or judgment; it does not understand *self-loathing* or *insecurity*. It uses an entirely different lexicon than we do, one that assumes its own naturalness and right to exist.

When we allow ourselves to be open to the call of this animal within, we realize that we desire a glorious stretch of our spirits. A wolf does not doubt, question, or restrain her body and inherent nature, she will howl for connection, for excitement, for soothing, for loneliness, for togetherness, for boredom, for longing, for lust, for beauty, and for no other reason at all other than that it just feels so good. She has the confidence to assert her desires and hunt down what she needs.

The knowing of confidence within our animal bodies begins with tuning in to them. When we wake up the body, the mind wakes up. When the mind wakes up, then the spirit wakes up. When the mind-body-spirit is awake, you finally have the ability to act with autonomy, which is the root of feminine confidence.

I recommend that once you have read through all of the body area sections, choose one area to focus on for three to four weeks. This may seem like a long time, but in my own experimentations, I have found that in order to release my guardedness I needed to offer myself weeks of intentional engagement. These body areas need the gentle repetition of presence and care.

My intention is for you to form new habits in your body. Giving yourself the time you need to form these habits reinforces a sturdier, enduring form of confidence in you. As Charles Duhigg writes in *The Power of Habit*, "Although each habit means relatively little on its own, over time, the meals we order, what we say to our kids each night, whether we save or spend, how often we exercise, and the way we organize out thoughts and work routine have enormous impacts on our health, productivity, financial security, and happiness."[12]

Internal Compass: The Pelvis

When we feel our feet to be like roots, energetically stretching themselves ever deeper into the black interior of the Earth, we are a little steadier, a little less windblown in our lives. And it is from this place that the energy of our attention can begin to run up the thick columns of our legs, our powerful, elephant-like thighs, moving toward the country of our pelvic well.

Our pelvis resembles a set of great boney antlers that have fallen off the head of a stag and lodged deeply in our muddy earth, raised tips attuned to the sky. Between the bony protuberances of our hips rests a wide fertile valley, a place where all the creative creatures within us can come to drink, eat, dance, and be nourished.

For ease of understanding and orientation, let us orient with the bony structures, then move through the tissues, then consider the energetics. Upholding a more three-dimensional viewpoint will allow us to better understand movement and flow through the entire pelvic bowl.

Begin by thinking of the pelvic area as an open space whose edges trace the pelvic floor and public bone. Then place your hands on the crests of your hip bones and feel their sturdy presence. Slide your hands on either side of your lower abdomen and lower back, just staying present with what lives here.

This space contains an array of busy viscera: digestive, urinary, and reproductive organs. In women, these reproductive organs engage in complex interactions with the rest of their bodies. The pelvic space is unusual in that it holds matter (digestive waste, fluids, even growing babies) while also being able to move substances down and out. It knows when to hold and when to release.

If we take our explorations past the bony structure, past the physical organs, all the way to the energetics of this space, we will find the archetype of the Artist-Visionary waiting there. In fact this space, between the sacrum ("sacred") and the pelvis ("vessel"), or *sacred vessel,* is considered a well of divine power.

Coach and author LiYana Silver describes the pelvic bowl as the seat of an aspect of our psyche that she calls the *Oracle.* The Oracle always knows what we are truly passionate about, what feels meaningful, what moves us in life. In *Feminine Genius,* Silver explains: "Your Oracle not only creates life, it also brings meaning to your life. Your Oracle is not only an organ of pleasure, but also an organ of truth. Your Oracle, it turns out, is not an appendage that you tow around like a dinghy on a ship, but an engine, steering wheel, compass, and headquarters, all in one."[13] The pelvis is the home of our joy in creating something out of nothing. This is the holy center of our bodies where our babies and other creative seeds are planted.

I have spent much of my life learning from the pelvic space. Diagnosing and assessing through the *hara,* or abdomen, has been an integral part of my work as an acupuncturist. After putting my hands on the lower abdomens of thousands of women, I have observed two basic patterns. In the most simplistic of terms, as women we are either tightened down (which could also present as numbed out or shut off) or empty/weakened (no or little energy lighting up this area).

Most women have moved through their lives never connecting with or seeing the need to pay attention to this area of their bodies. So often we have no female guides to school us in the amazing capacities of the female body and so we remain oblivious or anesthetized to the potential of this remarkable area. There can be a lasting deadness here—a certain immobilization.

Years and years of avoiding pregnancy and making conscious attempts to ignore even the existence of our reproductive organs and pelvic bowl can cause a certain dullness to set in. Women have fewer reasons or opportunities to attend to their cycles and signs in modern culture. More and more time is spent in some false regulation of them, our birth control pills acting as a clever cloak. Hushed sensations replace clear communication—the voice of our inner knowing quieted by energy weakness, depletion, lack of connection, or disassociation.

But the disconnect that resides here is not always from exhaustion, not always from picking up more weight and placing it on top of what we already carry. No, sometimes we have been unconsciously clenching so hard that nothing turns on here anymore. We have been sucking in and training our bellies so militantly that now they only speak the language of a white-knuckled grip. Finally tuning in, we may begin to see how our pelvic space has become its own locked gateway of unconscious tension, pain, and stress, keys nowhere to be found.

This area of the body can begin to list away from us, feeling more remote with every passing year. We are taught to birth our creations through the schedules and agendas of the outer world instead of connecting with the inner rhythm of our own bodies.

Reconnection insistently begins with an acknowledgement of the power and life force that resides here. Yes, I am interested in the chemistry, the soft tissue and the organs that run through here (and all of their interrelatedness) but what I am most curious about is the strength and flow of the energy that lives here. Is there a spark of aliveness? A container by nature, the irony of the pelvic bowl is that it contains the source of our life force and creativity, but it also ends up being a dumping ground for our blocks, an unconscious place to stash away unresolved trauma and fear.

Many systems of Indigenous medicine around the world understand the core energy that resides in the lower abdomen, which is also known as the *sea of qi*. The sixth-century B.C.E. Taoist teacher

Lao Tzu describes in his scriptures that this is where "essence and spirit are stored . . . related to regeneration, sexual energy, menstruation, and semen."[14] Basically, the pelvis is considered to be the storehouse of our life force, like a special holding area for strength and stamina.

How do we awaken body areas that have been in long, persistent slumber? How can we better connect with the power and confidence that wants to grow from our pelvic space?

Begin with touch. Place your hands on your lower abdomen. Be curious and listen.

Learn to breathe from your belly as a way to spark life force here. Most of us breathe from the upper lobes of our lungs, sometimes even up into our clavicles. The sensation that is generated in the body from this short shallow breathing is one of anxiety and constraint.

Begin with abdominal breathing. With your mind's eye placed a couple of inches below your navel, on the inhale let your abdomen expand. On the exhale let your abdomen relax. In the beginning, this practice may feel forced or unnatural, but we all came into this life with this skill. As peaceful sleeping babies, we were naturally able to belly breathe with ease.

Belly breathing has been found to lower blood pressure and heart rate, as well as to decrease the level of stress hormones circulating in the body.[15] When we practice breathing in this way, it is a restorative balm to the nervous system, relaxing and soothing our spirits.

Energy rides on the movement of the breath. Imagine your breath moving downwards, enlivening and awakening your pelvic space. Let it tune you in to any unconscious clenching or tensing that you have been doing here, stuffing down any past feelings. Imagine the breath expanding, nourishing, circulating your life force here. There is an elemental confidence that lives here too—it acts as a continually bubbling spring that rises up from your rich inner grounds, flowing upwards and out into the world.

Calling upon the wisdom of the Artist-Visionary, take some time to explore these pelvic reconnection exercises and journal questions:

- *What if, reduced to the size of a fairy, you climbed inside your pelvic space? If you were to roam the mountains of your hips and roll down the slot canyons of your tender insides, what would you find there? What might you be holding here in terms of tension, emptiness, or emotion? When you really tune in, what does this area of your body have to tell you?*

- *Create a habit of regularly connecting with your pelvic bowl. When you get into bed at night lay a hand on your belly and begin a practice of abdominal breathing. You can also do self-massage or use heat on your abdomen as a way to further relax and connect.*

- *Ongoingly check in with how you are holding your lower belly during the daytime. The cultural programming to have flat abs lingers with us still. Most of us have been sucking in our stomachs our entire lives, so that we now unconsciously clench the muscles of our lower abdomen and pelvic bowl even when we have no need to do so. As an antidote to ongoing subtle tension, regularly visualize this area as lit up, like a relaxed, radiant white globe of light, shining brightly. Use the energy generated from this light to let a sense of confidence naturally radiate.*

Bone Trunk: The Spine

Along the upper portion of your sacrum lies an important meeting point with the rest of your spine. The thirty-three short, irregular bones of the spine stack up, one atop the other, protecting and housing your precious spinal cord and spinal nerves. Any practitioner of yoga understands the importance of sun salutations, making a physical prayer to the sun while bending and rising to flush out the spine's fluid over and over again. This elongated trunk of pearly white is designed to be massaged and circulated in this way, as it rules over the health and longevity of the nervous system.

The standing people, the teachers we call *trees,* are constantly showing us the meaning of backbone. The conifers are a particularly good example of uprightness, their arms stretched to the sky and their feet reaching toward the belly of the Earth. They speak of quiet integrity, the good of discipline, the internal fortitude that comes from energy flowing through a strong posture.

It is for this reason that there is a tradition of placing wooden ridgepoles within Tibetan *stupas* (dome-shaped shrines). The *sokshing* in a stupa is considered the sacred "spine" of a holy place. This word for the central support structure translates as "tree of life" because it is literally created from the trunk of a tree that has been carefully selected and harvested with the absolute intention of fulfilling its sacred purpose. This wood is treated and then elaborately carved, often with inner niches built into it to hold sacred texts, relics, or other precious objects. The pole's exterior is painted and decorated, and then the sokshing is placed back in the stupa vertically so that it can act as its divine spine while holding up the roof.[16]

The idea of the sokshing captured my imagination long ago. I loved the idea of sanctifying a building with the gift of a life force rod that had been infused with tree energy and layered with blessings whose energy waits to touch and interact with every visitor.

We, too, contain sacred spines. Just like the sokshing, our spines act as a pillar of vitality. The spine is the first structure that forms in a child's body during gestation, the initial diamond bits of our skeleton. Our spines allow for the expression of confident, upward-flowing energy, but they also allow us to be flexible, like a bending willow blown by the wind.

Due to the pressures of life, we can get sunken, our chests folding in, our shoulders drooping forward, our necks and upper backs strained and stiff. If we're feeling drained or under attack, then our physical bodies will be a direct reflection of our emotional and spiritual depletion. How can we stand strong if our ridge poles are dried, brittle, and weak, and our inner energy has been entirely consumed? No matter how much we might try to fake it, it's virtually impossible to feel true confidence on occasions when we are deeply weary.

We know that trees whose trunks have not grown vertically can become susceptible to breakage from disease, storms, or snow. We too feel stronger on all levels when our posture is upright and strong, reflecting our healthy will.

There is also something essentially stabilizing to our psyche and physical form when our feet are strongly connecting with the ground and our spines erect. Our feet want to spread and push, the intricate bones of our toes wide open and elongated, a sturdy lattice work for standing and walking. Our primary connection point to the Earth, our feet are one of the most underappreciated, overused areas of the human body. They work tirelessly, taking all the weight of our ambition and relentless doings.

Feeling our feet firmly on the ground or the floor is the very beginning, the essential starting point of so many awareness and body practices. When we attune to them, they ask us to perceive how we intentionally connect, forming communion with stone, with holy dirt, with wooden floorboards, or whatever surface we are grounding into.

A certain relaxation takes over when we can find this sturdy still point where we are lengthening to the sky—it is the opposite of forced stiffness. There is a reason that the term *Mountain pose* is found in the yogic tradition of India. What does it mean to embody the energy of a mountain, steady and patient? There is inherent confidence in feeling so settled. There is no artificial pumping up, sticking out the chest, or inflating ourselves in an overly forced way.

Mountain stance also feels androgynous. It embodies a balance of masculine and feminine energy, both of which reside within all of us. It connects the energy from Father Sky above, the cosmic flow, with the energy from Mother Earth below, the primal giver of life, and it melds them, with perfect alchemy, at the heart center.

Our Inner Healer energy has some ideas on how we can connect with and take care of this confidence column in the body. Here are a few more questions and suggestions to help you reflect on the confidence that runs through your spine:

- *Touch into the energy and message of the bones of your spine. What do they have to tell you about your will, inner strength, striving, and physical stamina? What message of health (or health challenge) do they express, and how does that reflect your confidence?*

- *Our spines are meant to move in every direction, every day. The spaces in between your vertebrae are meant to be opened and cleansed with a regular infusion of blood. They are meant to be rinsed out through the circulation of your life force. They are not meant to sit in the same position all day long, turning into one stiff, fused block of concrete. Contemplate how your spine moves or doesn't move each day. How could more movement in your spine free up more flow and life force in your body?*

- *Become the devoted, respectful student of a tree. Ask some gentle giant that lives near you for guidance on how to live. Always moving with the wind and the flow of life, while enduringly watchful, what does this tree have to show you about a natural, unwavering confidence?*

Love Chalice: The Heart Space

Flowing upward along the spine, we come to a swirling pool of energy within the center of the chest. This is the confidence that surges through the powerhouse of a heart whose arms are wide open. What could be more daring, more stirring, than the atomic flash of a love unrestrained by all our hurts, traumas, insecurities, and modes of self-protection? To know love as the ultimate unifying force across cultures and continents is the true medicine of the times we live in.

Learning the healthy boundaries of the heart is essential to navigating our way through the complexities of our world. If we are unable to discern when loving without boundaries has become detrimental to us, we can overidentify with or take on other people's pain—even the suffering of the entire world. In doing so, we can be left immobile and lost, leaving us thoroughly unhelpful to anyone, including ourselves. If we allow our hearts to become overworked and overheated, they end up shriveled pieces of fruit left out in the sunlight of limitless loving. But if we let our hearts grow too cold, their pink and bloody undulations slowly become replaced by the slow creep of stone.

Energy medicine maven Donna Eden calls the heart chakra (a major subtle energy center located in the center of the chest) the "chalice of both joy and sorrow." She concludes that it is an "underrated organ in modern cultures. While we are impressed with its resilience as a pump, most Indigenous cultures believe that thought originates in the heart, not the brain."[17]

For a long time, people of the West have underestimated the capabilities and true functioning of the heart. Even now, modern science is only just beginning to scratch the surface of what many ancient traditions have believed for thousands of years—that the heart is an access point for vast wisdom and intelligence. Buddhist teacher Jack Kornfield describes: "It is possible to speak with our heart directly. Most ancient cultures know this. We can actually converse with our heart as if it were a good friend. In modern life, we have become so busy with our daily affairs and thoughts that we have lost this essential art of taking time to converse with our hearts."[18]

The HeartMath Institute, a nonprofit organization that studies the "physiological mechanisms by which the heart and brain communicate," found that the activity of the heart influences our perceptions, emotions, intuition, and health.[19] In the early 1990s, they "were among the first to conduct research that not only looked at how stressful emotions affect the activity in the autonomic nervous system (ANS) and in the hormonal and immune systems, but also at the effects of emotions such as appreciation, compassion and care."[20] This is why the electromagnetic field around the heart, or the *heart brain,* is considered the seat of human wisdom in many eastern traditions.

Our understanding of our hearts needs to move way beyond their physicality to recognizing them as the suns they really are—center points in our own mini "solar systems." It is through our sun-hearts that we may experience our feeling selves, our insightful selves, our aware selves, our truth-perceiving selves. When we stop solely orienting from the kingdom of the rational, fix-it, solve-it, pin-it-down, and put-it-in-a-glass-case mentality, we can jump the chasm between *thinking* and *knowing.*

The repetitive messages that dominate our culture have taught us and reinforced the way of the mind, emphasizing the role of reasoning. But we also benefit from training more seriously in the way of the heart. In *The Pathwork of Self-Transformation,* psychic channel Eva Pierrakos describes what happens when you make room for the wisdom of the heart and your whole feeling self.

> *Through the gateway of feeling your weakness lies your strength.*
>
> *Through the gateway of feeling your pain lies your pleasure and joy.*
>
> *Though the gateway of feeling your fear lies your security and safety.*
>
> *Through the gateway of feeling your loneliness lies your capacity to have fulfillment, love, and companionship.*
>
> *Through the gateway of feeling your hopelessness lies true and justified hope.*
>
> *Through the gateway of accepting the lacks in your childhood lies your fulfillment now.*[21]

The softness we are seeking in ourselves rests on the essential, seemingly elusive practice of feeling into our feelings. The greatest work of the heart is to teach us about *availability*. How are we available (or not) to the challenging work of deep listening? How are we available (or not) to the uncomfortable, ugly feelings we might have about ourselves or others?

It is in this availability that we begin, shyly, to take the hand of *vulnerability*—to gently place our shields down on the ground and just let the breeze of open presence wash over us. This is to catch our first instinct when in conflict with others, which is to respond with defensiveness, frustration, or impatience. Because sometimes practicing kindness doesn't actually have anything to do with an actual act of kind doing. It could just mean showing up without weapons already drawn or without automatically trying to fix or change things.

We are deeply programmed against expressing this type of vulnerability or directing this kind of gentleness toward ourselves. We are conditioned to feel that vulnerability is too scary, fragile, unsafe, and, above all, an expression of weakness. The complete opposite of confidence.

But flowing through the veins of vulnerability is a pulsing, warrior-like courage. Because it is only through learning to bravely open our hearts to ourselves that we can learn to open them more easily to others. We have to become more aware of the aperture of our hearts, which has the capacity to narrow and widen like the great lens of a camera; it has an innate knowing of when to adjust itself to be a little more open, a little more closed.

Let a sun of confidence shine through your heart center, not just in the front across your clavicles but through the spaces between your ribs, radiating out in all directions, even through your back. So often we wear a rusted carapace on our backs, the turtle shell of all our protection, all our holding. Yet another shield. When the imbalances and weakness of the pelvis and lower abdomen are reflected upward, the heart center eventually begins to show signs of collapse. With shoulders rounded forward, pectoral muscles tightened, upper back muscles lengthened, we become stooped like our grandmothers before our time.

By its very nature, the heart center wants to spread, wants to know the opposite of slumping forward. It wants to pull aliveness from all around us and then radiate it out in every direction. It yearns for long-held back bends and opportunities to study those hanging luminaries of stars in the sky. It craves enormous breaths, bouquets of clear air, and fierce, unyielding expansion.

The Space Dancer wants you to walk the edge of what feels contradictory about opening your heart, to discover what is daring and strong about vulnerability. Feel into the health of your heart center by reflecting and journaling on these questions:

- *Begin every day with the audacious and authentic act of inviting in the worthiness of your feelings by asking the question: "How am I feeling right now?" Name a feeling and describe it in colors, flavors, textures, and temperature to yourself. With your hand on your heart, explore if you can be hurt, or lost, or grieving, or overwhelmed and still be available.*

- *Mentally tune in to the physicality of how you hold your chest, ribcage, upper back, and shoulders. How does this reflect how sturdy or worn out you feel in your life? How does rolling your shoulders back and spreading open through your chest shift your sense of presence and confidence?*

- *Use five minutes of visualization to soak yourself into the medicine of love, to give thanks for the wonderful, hardworking, ever-beating heart in your chest. Feel the energy of love running deep through the center of your torso, letting it become a growing, radiating, expanding love-light.*

Soul Mirrors: The Eyes

Imagine the ghostly way that a jaguar stalking its prey moves through a forest. It is so aware of its surroundings that its every sense tingles and sparks as the silent pads of its paws touch the Earth floor. Although not nearly so well adapted, our senses are also always on, ready to ignite.

Each of our senses is precious and essential to fully exploring our worlds. Our ears, noses, and mouths are orifices of delight, reporting the details of their discoveries—sounds, scents, and flavors—to our ever-expectant brains. But it is our eyes that are the hued reflectors of our souls, revealing our essence outwardly. They crease, they swell, they drip, they laugh, and they carelessly divulge our feelings.

According to traditional Chinese medicine, there is a way of understanding someone's overall vitality and mental clarity by looking into their eyes: assessing their *shen*. Shen is a person's natural radiance, which can be seen in the eyes. It can also refer to a person's "inner spirit, awareness, consciousness, mental faculties."[22]

When our eyes are dull or shrouded, they speak to the heaviness and stagnation of our life force. But when our eyes are bright, they reflect our curiosity, vitality, and flow. Eyes are the truth-tellers of the face, honestly revealing how we are genuinely feeling.

Looking deeply into another being's eyes is as primal as it gets. In *The Moon by Whale Light*, Diane Ackerman portrays her experience of swimming with right whales in Patagonia in a protected bay on their way to the rich feeding grounds of Antarctica. She describes the majesty of having one of the whales swim within two feet of her, turning its head to reveal an "eye much like a human eye. I looked directly into her eye, and she looked directly back at me, as we hung in the water, studying each other. . . . The only emotion I sensed was her curiosity. That shone through her watchfulness, her repeated turning toward us, her extreme passivity, her caution with flippers and tail. Apparently, she was doing what we were—swimming close to a strange, fascinating life-form, taking care not to frighten or hurt it."[23]

When that "dark, plum-like eye" fixed on her, Ackerman drank of the deep intelligence and immense inquisitiveness of the whale. Unlike whales, many other animals, among them dogs and gorillas, make direct eye contact with human or animal strangers with extreme caution. The forwardness of eye-to-eye interaction can be considered a show of aggression and intimidation, igniting a primitive flight-or-fight instinct.

The same response to direct eye contact is true, albeit to a lesser degree, for humans. Weak eye contact is an immediate sign to another person that you are feeling wary, insecure, or generally uncertain of yourself or the situation. Weak eye contact can also be a default, compensatory posture used by those not wanting to seem overly aggressive, intense, or intimidating. Many women also unconsciously find themselves looking away, not wanting to be blamed for being too direct or seemingly coming on "too strong."

Of course, we don't always want to reveal what we are thinking or feeling. Because our eyes expose our stress levels, they convey our honest feelings beyond the lies of an upturned mouth or appeasing words. Our pupils, in particular, are constantly adjusting and making changes without our knowledge. As human sociobiology expert Desmond Morris, D. Phil., describes: "The pupils cannot lie because we have no conscious control over them."[24] This is why professional poker players wear dark sunglasses; they are looking to cover up any involuntary changes in their eyes that might be too revealing of their emotional state.

In his work as an optometrist, Jacob Israel Liberman, O.D., Ph.D., author of *Luminous Life,* has documented how when people work from the "push," or from taking a more strenuous, intense approach to their lives, their pupils shrink and the light in their eyes becomes dimmer. Engaging in our lives with this pushing energy restricts our inner light.

Liberman describes how our "potential as human beings is hinged on the subtle balance between striving and thriving."[25] When people are working with ease and remembering to breathe, the eyes instantaneously respond with an expansion of the pupils and a filling of light. It is some sort of light feedback loop, for "happiness allows us to see, remember, and understand more, expanding the size of the window through which we see the world."[26] Having a sense of tunnel vision, shrinking your field of perception, literally collapses your overall awareness and engagement with life.

According to a study reported in the *Journal of Experimental Psychology,* when we look deeply into another person's eyes while conversing, the pupils of both individuals spontaneously synchronize.[27] The eyes are unique in this way: they are both *projective* and *reflective*. But how frequently do we give rapt attention to one another this way, really pulling in and allowing ourselves to be washed over by someone's eyes?

It is worth the uncomfortable experiment.

Vast kaleidoscopes of expression, a flecked mosaic of colors we might not have thought could live in eyes can be found there: glowing fire embers, specks of mica, flaxy grasses, and sea storm grays.

The eyes are a gateway that draws us in, reminding us that our eyes are part of all other "eyes" in the universe: the eyes of an animal, the eye of a dahlia, the eye of a storm, the eye of a faraway nebula, the eye within the whorl of a mollusk, and the eye painted on a Luna moth's wing. Our eyes hold more mystery than we realize, acting as an entry point to some direct connection to the blinking eyes of the mystic stars themselves.

Good eye contact does not need to feel intimidating. Instead, it can come from a perspective of being attentive and engaged. Calling on the Artist-Visionary as an invoker of curiosity and creativity, here are a few more ways for you to explore confidence through the realm of the eyes:

- *Look into the eyes of someone you think you know well with a renewed sense of wonder and attention. Is your immediate instinct to pull away? If you can stay with a relaxed interest, slowly describe the color of the person's eyes to yourself. And then don't just stop at the color, get really specific about the shade: Are the eyes sugar-caramel brown, sea glass blue and so forth? Then, focus on the shape of the eyes and how clear their whites are. How far or close together are the eyes?[28] What do the pupils tell you about the person's sense of ease or stress?*

- *Alternately imagine that you are breathing and smiling through your eyes. Most of us breathe in very shallow, irregular rhythms, but when you "breathe" through your eyes, they light up and shine outwards. Tune in to how your face, posture, and entire body changes when you do this. How does this impact your sense of confidence and how do others around you respond?*

Pelvis as a fertile valley, backbone as a life force trunk, heart as a sun of availability, eyes as reflectors of truth, these are some of the many places that confidence inherently lives in us, potent parts of our personal geography.

Sit still with your body. Hear it speaking. Respect its voice. What does it tell you about body as foreign, body as home, body as complex, body as gift? What does the secret life of your body want you to know about how you have lived? What openness wants to be expressed within the vortices of your tension? Yes, there is spaciousness, even there.

May a more conscious sense of embodiment be present with you now.

May being awake in your flesh provide an ever-open gateway to remembering your feminine confidence.

May you believe in the shocking holiness of your body, that you are thunder made flesh, meant to roll us over with your beauty.

May all the places that you have become numbed out, shut off, or compartmentalized feel reconnected.

May you no longer need to ask permission, may your body no longer speak in apologies, may the voice of your wants sing loudly, and may you really listen.

CHAPTER FIVE

Sacred Initiations

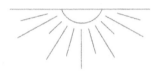

"Do not be dismayed by the brokenness of the world. All things break. And all things can be mended. Not with time, as they say, but with intention. So go. Love intentionally, extravagantly, unconditionally. The broken world waits in the darkness for the light that is you."[1]

—L. R. KNOST

Every creature on this planet knows what it means to *return*. No matter where you come from, no matter where you live, there is some route you know as intimately as the wrinkles of your own palm. You have traveled through this place—smooth asphalt, forested path, or cracked sidewalk—so many times that you unconsciously anticipate its bends and curves like the tossing of some rough sleep. The same humble landmarks, the same red or green lights, the same trickster potholes have greeted you again and again.

That to Which We Return

What do we return to again and again as an act of unthinking magnetism? Whether it is a physical space, a person, a thought pattern, or a holy habit, what has become buried in the arch of the body and in the ether of the psyche through the power of its repetition? What turns us over, the gradual insistence of erosion, the way water hits the Earth, the way time hits our faces, and the way a sculptor hits stone?

The dusty cellars of our minds are constantly being shaped by our repetition. It is here that we store thick encyclopedias of stories, crafted by what we bring our attention to again and again. The wizardry of these stories rests in our seductive retelling of them—in the words and images—as much as in the feelings they evoke.

Even those of us who were born after the heyday of CDs can still relate to them as a metaphor to understand how a story plays out in our minds. The tiny grooves and bumps etched into the surface of a disc hold the information of that particular story, and as the laser of our mental "CD player" passes over those same grooves again and again, we grind that story deeper into our subconscious mind.

Activist and author Rebecca Solnit explains: "We tell ourselves stories that save us and stories that are the quicksand in which we thrash and the well in which we drown, stories of justification, of accursedness, of luck and star-crossed love, or versions clad in the cynicism that is at times a very elegant garment. . . . Not a few stories are sinking ships, and many of us go down with these ships even when the lifeboats are bobbing all around us."[2]

Now we really like to hang tight to these kinds of stories, the ones that involved shock, fear, trauma, grief, disappointment, and betrayal. It is kind of amazing how much effort we put into replaying of these past, broken accounts of our lives compared to the energy required to peer into the unknown of creating new ones.

The reason we hang on to stories of trauma so strongly is because our brains are programmed to protect us. When something bad happens, we want to make sure that it *never* happens again. We are evolutionarily motivated to protect ourselves this way, or as the neurobiologist Rick Hanson describes it, we are Velcro to the negative and Teflon to the positive.[3]

There is some intelligence in this, right? It makes sense that we wouldn't want to get hurt in the same ways again. The trouble with this tendency is that as ever-evolving human beings, many of these stories we repeat just plain aren't accurate anymore. They are a mirage of truth, seemingly sturdy in their retelling and then dissolving into a misty haze upon deeper examination. But we are unconsciously driven to keep playing those same old familiar CDs because it feels easier and safer. They offer us a view of the world that makes it seem predictable and known.

With honest inquiry we often come to realize that many of the stories that regulate our actions were created by our childhood selves, at a vulnerable stage in our development when we had a lot less control over our lives. As children, the majority of our stories were based in a few very primary fears.

- Fear of no love
- Fear of death or annihilation
- Fear of abandonment
- Fear of being ostracized or separated from our clan

These are our deepest motivating fears in life, and they are planted in our will to survive. Exposing these foundational worries allows us to make contact with our scared younger self who created them and to soothe her into seeing her everyday reality as it really is.

Because we no longer need to apply the stories of our early life to the everyday truths of our current life, this may be a good time to ask: Who were you before these CDs started playing in the first place?

What was your essence? I would contend that each of us has a spark of genuine confidence within her that has never changed—it just got besieged by all the other noises in her head. Because when life gets all filled up with our drama stories, there is very little space left for our soul's intention story.

Deepening our tracking skills and remembering our jaguar-like senses, we can make contact with the self-assured girl that lives within each of us still. Perhaps she can offer insights into any core confidence wounds and the circumstances in which they were incurred. Imprints from these wounds from an earlier stage of your life may well be influencing your current ideas about perfection, failing, risk-taking, pleasing, self-acceptance, and more.

The truth is that most of us come to know our confidence through experiences of the unconventional, the unpleasant, and the unwanted—times when the wind gets knocked out of our lungs and we must fight the urge to panic, humbly waiting for the breath to return again. This kind of unshakeable confidence is learned through sacred initiations like flat-out failure, cycles of hardship, periods of questioning, feeling lost, hanging out in the dark, or even having a complete loss of trust in ourselves. We must have the courage to allow these hard things to inform us, break us, teach us, and change us for good.

Most women undergo some version of two sacred rites of passage that serve as confidence initiations.

- An initiation during the transition from girlhood to young womanhood, where her inherent feminine confidence is threatened. This is a time in life she may decide that it is safer to trade self-confidence for self-consciousness.
- An initiation through the crisis of making mistakes and discovering her imperfect self, which may lead to a loss of inner faith and lingering self-doubts.

These rites school us through a fierce engagement with challenge—
a teaching of how often we discover more in the darkness of our lives
than in the light. Sometimes it is only through periods of being cracked
wide open in the pitch-black that we can finally perceive the resilience,
self-loyalty, and hidden strength of our fierce feminine confidence.

The Machine

In most places, water lives within the constraints of its relationship
with the land. You will find it edged in and behaving itself within
shorelines, riverbanks, and coastal cliffs. But water in the Pacific
Northwest behaves differently. The barriers blend in these misty lands
and the rain is so fine and persistent that there seems no difference
between its liquid and gaseous states.

Really, it's not the rain herself, but the oppressive darkness of rainy
days that sometimes weighs on me. Waking in a tousled bed of gray
drizzle one morning, the actual drops of rain felt insignificant
compared to the heft of the clouds, which were massive and
foreboding as they loomed close to my head. Allowing myself a slower
than usual start and wanting to burrow into the bottom layers of the
bed, I began to unpack a freshly woven dream. Similar to the air
outside, the dream felt burdened. It had something to do with an old
contraption, comparable to one I might find in the graveyard of large
machines I grew up seeing in my father's engineering shop. I made the
following note of the dream in my journal.

*There are clunks and groans as the massive gears, well-oiled and worn,
turn with mechanical ease. The device is every shade of charcoal and tar,
lifeless and unconscious. The immense machine looms over her, a small
child, tiny and unmoving. There is a thick chain that links her cage to
somewhere in the bowels of the machine. The girl clutches herself in a tight*

ball, unaware that the door to her cage has slowly swung open. Something propels her to look up, to realize that she is free to go. She is terrified to move; it seems safer to stay put and pretend she doesn't see the exit.

But all of a sudden, she feels a warm, wet tongue on her hand, and she looks up to see the face of a young, excited puppy. The puppy continues to lick and nudge her until she has no choice than to get up and step out of the cage. She sees the brightness of the sky and the green grass of a vast lawn.

Outside, she starts to throw a ball for the puppy, and with each throw she feels something in her lighten. The puppy exudes an energy that is playful, loving, and loyal as it returns the ball again and again to her. Neither male nor female, it is a creature of pure youth. It holds the essence of trust and freedom.

It acts as some kind of reviver of possibility.

And it is in the repetition of every throw, the feeling in the action that reminds her there is something tucked in her pocket, humming. She digs into the crease of her pants, to find a treasure intricately folded over and put away long ago. Remembering it now, she discovers a hidden envelope of joy. As she peels at the layers of the envelope, there is an unfolding of paper wings, translucent and glassy.

Life wants to return to those wings, which had been hibernating passively for so long. They pulse with expanding grace, a push to awake. All of a sudden, a breeze moves through the grass and paper wings, and in an instant, hundreds of butterflies are dispersed into the sky. The girl feels her own heart travel with them, lost and found, uplifted by the unbounded beating of the many soul-bird wings.

This was one of those dreams that dawdle. Past breakfast, drifting out in random pauses throughout the day and into the next, its realness was unshakable. It seemed to lay a film of stickiness over me—especially the oppressive black energy of the machine at the beginning.

With further contemplation, I came to realize that this machine had the presence of an adult male. It contained the magnitude and impersonal nature of our larger cultural consciousness. It held the energy of the system that cannibalizes young girls and women, cutting off their voices and sacrificing their uniqueness.

The potency of the dream—the energy of the machine's bleak, unfeeling movements—points to how the invisible forces of our male-dominated culture begin to impress themselves on a young girl. Some imperceptible change occurs at the borderlands of puberty: a shift from being unbridled to something more tightly contained. Young girls at this age are like the shoots of plants in springtime: tender, precious, and very easily nibbled away. These shoots contain the leaves, the flowering stems, and buds needed for all further stages of development.

This reminds me of my young daughter's self-created description for her own slow-growing breasts, her "little rosebuds." The essence of this time period is so naturally radiant and brimming, yet dangerously easy to crush.

In *The Girl Within,* psychologist Emily Hancock describes in detail the magical threshold of eight or nine years old, a time when girls have yet to be imprinted with society's hidden messages. This is a time when her sense of self-mastery is unchallenged, a time to feel free, test boundaries, and live unapologetically. But just as puberty is beginning, a girl can become extremely aware of her so-called bodily imperfections and attune to a barrage of cultural cues to become a "young lady."

Hancock describes how "poised between the make-believe of preschool and the thrall of adolescence, a girl this age occupies an intermediate zone of childhood, an interim space between fantasy and reality that fosters creative self-ownership."[4]

And where does this girl go? What triggers this mysterious shift from being a spirited, playful, inherently self-assured individual to being self-punishing and self-restrained? When does self-confidence acquiesce to self-consciousness?

At some point around the time of puberty, the girl learns to slip on the heavy robe of the judge. Wooden gavel threateningly hung in midair, she is ready to strike herself down at any time. Her morphing body is endlessly analyzed, scrutinized within a combat zone of insecurity and increased risk. She may also learn the art of gossip, a means of putting others down in a pitiful attempt to lift herself up, becoming polished at balancing her fragile self atop of a pile of demeaned, limp bodies.

The shift in confidence at puberty that suddenly divides a girl from herself, splitting her psyche in two, is an initiation into a new identity. The outer girl-woman tersely moves on, fitting in and trying to belong within the constraints of society. Meanwhile the inner girl-child, possessing a soaring autonomy beyond cultural context, lays dormant as a seed with no water.

I can recall lying outstretched for hours in the long-cooled bathtub at my parents' house, staring at my form. My body at eleven seemed like a bizarre creature. Skin spreading, swelling, and moving. My emerging breasts were tiny lumps roused under a skin sheath. Hairs were growing like lone adult trees amid soft baby grasses.

There were changes afoot in my head as well. As if a little worm of doubt had crawled into my ear, nothing seemed right. One day my body wasn't changing fast enough to suit me: flat chest, no period. The next day I was feeling overwhelmed by my tiny breasts, shifting hips, tiny pimples. There was no in-between, change was either too fast or too slow.

Body as enemy. An unruly, foreign opponent. Its own sudden betrayal. This is a phenomenon many women can recall from this same age.

The glances and attention I got from others started to feel different to me too. I could not put it into words at that time, but I was sensing some new pressure, the weight of sly eyeballs. To feel preyed upon—by neighbors, by the bully at school, by the old man at the mall. The potential to be devoured seemed to lurk. I hadn't changed, yet somehow I was different. The momentum of the whole world was no longer with me. There was the odor of danger in the air. It seemed safest to grow smaller and smaller still.

Imperceptible.

Mute button pushed.

It is at the secret portal of this prepubescence that many girls begin to wonder, *To whom and what do I belong anymore?* The breathing of this and many other questions surface at this time. But self-doubt boils stronger once the bleeding actually starts.

Instead of being greeted with a mighty initiation ceremony honoring our full creative power and potential, menstruation becomes a passageway into great shame for too many of us. We are taught to hide it, sanitize it, even hate it. Instead of revering the dynamic genius of our wombs, we perceive the self-cleansing mechanisms of our fertile bodies as a disgusting failing.

As mature women, we are grown girls who are looking to follow the lines in our lives back through time, back to the period when we were wounded and lost touch with our power—just when we should have been stepping into it. We can look back on the grim milestone when our voices went mute and find healing. Following the lines back is a journey to reconnect with the spirited, autonomous force deep inside us. Many of us long to hold her close and invite her to inform and guide our lives again.

I invite you to do so now.

Emily Hancock describes the *girl within,* and the deep truth she possesses, as the key to unlocking the essential female self. This girl is "competitive in the proper spirit, she is driven by mastery—not to dominate and seize power over others but to grasp the mysteries and challenges of the world herself."[5]

Reconnecting with the girl within gives a grown woman like you access to a limitless, self-governing landscape where she can reclaim her authenticity and sense of belonging.

If you began to "pour some water" on any dormant seeds of prowess within you, what would that look like for you? How might you revive it today? I felt the girl within me awakening in my dream of the machine, slowly at first—coming to her senses increasingly with every throw of that ball. For me, she signifies the healthiness of being a girl-child, beautifully free in herself.

As she gets ready to unfold the butterflies, my inner girl has a palpable sense of transformation. From her cold cage of restriction, she moves into a space of liberation big enough for her to fly.

Making contact with the girl within helps us to better understand the nature and history of our confidence wounds and what is needed for their healing. Calling in the intuitive wisdom of the Inner Healer, take out your journal and creatively explore the following questions.

- *What was your rite of passage like in your transition of girlhood to young womanhood? If you could redo this sacred initiation time, imagine what kind of ritual or experience you might recreate to baptize yourself into a lifelong sense of confidence?*

- *Becoming curious about the inherent confidence of the young girl within you, feel into her energy and wisdom. Write about any dormant seeds of autonomy from that time of girlhood that want to bloom within you now.*

Old Skin

Injuries to our confidence are at the meaty center of a conglomeration of issues that keep so many of us stuck in our lives: fearing to go for the big, courageous leaps we want to take, inhibiting our ability to contribute all we have, or scared to receive all that we say we want. They keep us in the job we outgrew two years ago or the relationship that is comfortably stale. Those early confidence wounds show up in all sorts of unexpected locations of adulthood, firmly tethering us in place, holding us back individually and collectively.

Many women don't realize that their confidence took leave long, long ago and that they have been living on hushed vapors of self-esteem ever since. But then there is a trigger—perhaps a divorce, an illness, a job loss, or a sudden fall out with a friend—and a confidence emergency ensues, seemingly out of nowhere. It is only then that the reality of their unexamined confidence— the truth that was waiting for them below the shallows—rises to the surface of their awareness.

I lost my mojo a few years back. This time there was no huge event, no obvious trauma or reason for it leaving. It felt like this spark of power within me just slipped out the bedroom window while I was sleeping. It took a while for me to even recognize its disappearance, to realize there was some sort of catastrophe underway.

Slowly I began to notice that I felt less guided and sure of myself at work and less self-assured in my relationships with others. I seemed plagued by worry and self-doubt; it was as if my inner critic had tripled in size and was stomping around in my head, taking up space and screaming at me through a megaphone.

I would like to say that this was a brief and passing phase, as sometimes happens. I kept waiting for it to mysteriously move along on its own. After a few months, I started to feel like something was really wrong, but I didn't know what to do about it. I felt as if I was getting some message downloaded from above, but I was sitting on the damn decoder.

Now, where did I put that thing?

About a year into my crisis, feeling stripped-down and fragile, I realized the painful, blinding truth: I had never really felt that confident from the get-go. Deep self-doubt had been plaguing me for years, and at some point, I had tried to just tune out its presence. Hence, I was confident on the outside—my outer mask was nicely polished. On the inside, I was an anxious, tense mess.

During that time, an image started to reveal itself to me: I felt as if I was inching my way through a dark cave, surprised by every sudden puddle and passing squeak. I was pissed to have to be there at all, and, by the way, when was someone going to light a match? This kind of stubborn and semi-resistant searching persisted for a lot longer than I care to admit.

But at some point, it dawned on me—

I have not actually lost anything.

I am just in a period of change.

There was no inner hole to fill, no lacking special sauce, no key to fit a lock.

I was just shedding skins. Lots of old skins. I had become ready to outgrow multiple layers of outdated thinking and behavior (although I didn't know it yet), and instead of needing to be on some search, I was just in the process of a transformation. This is also where it dawned on me that orienting from a sense of self-tenderness would serve me a lot better than the repetitive foot-stamping of hard-headed resistance.

As I continued to fumble my way through the dark, I invited the spirit and essence of Snake into my life to teach me about letting go of what I no longer needed.

Questions arose, such as: *What else needs to die during this time?*

In the wild, snakes molt as they are growing. Rubbing their noses against the ground, they expertly slither their way out of their long, thin shells, sloughing off any parasites in the process. Yes, I was growing emotionally *and* wanting to be rid of some very unhelpful thought patterns. I was also learning to become more comfortable in the dark, pressing my belly up against the Earth, just resting for a while in the empty unknown.

In Elam, one of the last ancient strongholds of Goddess reverence, which was located in the modern region of southwestern Iran, the snake was a symbol of feminine wisdom that was often depicted in bronze castings and pottery. In this small land, lying in the Zagros Mountains between the Caspian Sea and the Persian Gulf, the fertility symbol of the Tree of Life always came with a coiling serpent.

In reflecting on this symbol, I also asked: *What wants to be born in me at this time?*

The spirit of Snake in western culture has been seen as intricately connected to the deep, primal energy of our life force. Perhaps because snakes stay alive while shredding something dead. The symbol of a serpent encircling a staff was used in the cult of the Greek demigod Asclepios, associated with healing and medicine. Nonvenomous snakes also casually inhabited the floors of Asclepeion hospitals, symbolizing the dual nature of sickness and health, life and death, ever encircling each other.[6]

As part of my healing process, Snake wanted me to learn how to use my energy authentically and to better understand where I was drawing it from. This has been, and continues to be, a huge, repetitive lesson for me over the course of my life. After so many years in service to others, I am *still* learning how to be in service to myself.

With so many skins on my soul shed, I touched the raw, fresh layer underneath. I practiced applying healing salves of self-devotion, mothering and tending to myself as my own lover and medicine woman.

With so many skins on my soul shed, I looked into my own eyes to ask: *What is at the heart of your confidence wound?*

And I would ask you the same: What are the entrenched ways in which you continue to believe that you need to be different from who you really are?

Are there any sneaky methods by which you continue to source your confidence outside yourself?

These questions continue the healing, shedding process, letting it feel organic instead of frustrating. I wonder how many pounds and pounds of skin will be shed in my single life, floating husks to be taken back to the Earth. For when these periods of wandering through the dark of uncertainty come for me (you know they will), I aspire to let this darkness be my ally.

Allowing ourselves to be broken open to life—even through crisis—can temporarily feel like a loss of time and space, confusing up and down, ego and outcome, while holding us in the black belly of something so much bigger. But there is some naturalness to the process of this initiation; it seems to eat and sleep on its own time. If we are brave enough to let it take us, we will be freer in the end for it. If we can find the courage we might ask: What gifts want to be brought back from the underworld?

For it is only in the ashen intensity of angry storm clouds that we have a brighter perspective on sudden patches of pale blue sky. Likewise, it is through traversing the dark that we find balance in the light. What if healing is less about getting closer to some perfect tranquility, free from difficulty and discomfort, and instead about becoming even more open to the painful beauty and complexity of your experience?

When life launches a great emptying, a hitting of rock bottom, a coming to your knees, it acts as a sifter; it allows everything that you thought you needed (and didn't) to fall away. Once the dust settles and you assess what remains, you realize that the only things you really need are those very things that can never be taken away.

In the most vulnerable of moments, you are called to choose even more shakiness, more trust, more openness, more exposure of your soft belly and tender heart. Writing coach and word diva Jeannette LeBlanc donates some beautiful thoughts here: "This is what it feels like to be brilliantly achingly alive. Alive in the shatter. Alive in the empty. . . . This is what it is to belong to things we cannot possibly understand. This is what it is to trust in the terrifying wisdom of our own becoming."[7]

Calling on the queen of navigating the dark, the Space Dancer wants you to trust in your becoming. Take out your journal and explore these questions.

- *Reflect on any times you went through a sacred initiation or confidence crisis. What did you learn from this experience that has changed and morphed you still?*

- *Buddhist author and teacher Pema Chödrön describes: "Only to the extent that we expose ourselves over and over to annihilation can that which is indestructible be found in us."[8] What have you found to be indestructible inside you, despite everything?*

Love and Mistake-Making

Motherhood is one long initiation process. But this tiring baptism is not for women alone—children, too, grow through the trials of difficulty and change.

They are not meant to come through this rite-of-passage untouched. Not just mentally or emotionally unscathed, but also in the everyday physical way. Bumps, bruises, scrapes, and an array of other injuries are how we learn as kids. It is kind of illuminating and unrelenting all at once. It is the job of the child to fail constantly and yet keep on trying. The child does not question any of this, she just keeps on getting up, keeps on going, keeps on growing.

The child's passage feels mirrored in the truth that it is also impossible to escape the mighty rite of motherhood unbroken. That we are not meant to, either. That it is our job as parents to fail and yet to keep learning and loving constantly. In many ways, the mother and the child are engaging in some sort of enigmatic spiral dance, swirling in a stew of unfathomable love, frustration, love, exhaustion, love, mistake-making, love, and so on.

Like many new parents, I was loaded down with an overstuffed storage container of assumptions, false ideas, and good intentions. I was convinced I would not make any of the mistakes my parents made. I would do mothering *perfectly*.

I held this fantasy that my dear infant daughter and I would lie out on the lawn together in the summer, and she would goo and gaa and make pretty eyes at me. She would be like all the babies that I seemed to see around, angelic and content (clearly, I did not know a lot of babies).

Without even knowing anything about children, you can sniff out what happened next. It's like that predictable moment in a movie where you can sense that it is not going to end well. My entire world turned into a snow globe replica of itself, and somehow, through the power of this tiny human, that snow globe was turned upside down and shaken vigorously.

Without knowing it, I had entered a sacred initiation.

First of all, my daughter was born in the dark of winter. There was no summer grass or blanket on the lawn, but a thick sky blanket of rain clouds that seemed to rest permanently about five feet from my head. Brief lingerings of calm and contentment seemed only to come when she was nursing, which she seemed to do as if from a very thin straw. This meant long stretches of napping and nursing with the waking periods filled with unrelenting crying. There was so much crying (and the nagging sensation, *Something is wrong, is it supposed to be like this?*) that by two years of age she was unofficially diagnosed with sensory-processing disorder.

This revelation happened quite by accident. Due to some respiratory plague she had caught while traveling, I took my daughter to a pediatrician in a different state. While completing a general intake form, the practitioner gathered some overall constitutional information to figure out the best course of treatment. As she was asking us questions, you could sense some sort of suspicion creeping into her questions.

"She only calms down when you are pushing her as hard as you can in the swing?

"It takes her an hour to transition from the living room to the bathroom to her bedroom every night?

"The slightest textures bother her skin, and she hates being restricted by her car seat?

"How many outbursts does she have in a day?!"

It felt like by complete accident this lovely woman saved our lives. She mentioned the possibility of sensory-processing issues and a light bulb turned on in the pitch black. It gave me a desperately needed, rectifying switch in perspective. Of course, my dear one didn't mean to be hardheaded, extra difficult, exhausting, and demanding, she just didn't feel comfortable in her own skin.

This was my inception into the deep waters of parenting. Like a clumsy cannonball, however, it was a high height to fall from. There was no way to make it through that much crying and not feel the heavy, penetrating ache of failure, like a constant companion.

I did not have what it would take to make my child happy.

More than a decade later, it still produces a visceral reaction in my heart to feel the pain of wishing I could have sailed through those waters more skillfully. The grief of that very imperfect start is still slightly warm to the touch.

It feels as though I entered this learning from the backdoor. I thought that if I worked hard enough, swaddled, rocked, bounced, fed, changed, hugged, held, and loved enough, failure would have no space to exist. But failure still got in there somehow, that tricky bastard. I had a fixed mindset on how motherhood was supposed to go, and the reality was vastly different.

It is the snare of perfectionism that deceives us into thinking everything must look and feel a certain way. This trap strips us from finding and experiencing the magical texture and unnamed color of the present moment. It also steals our ability to stick with the sacred ugliness of our feelings, to make space and room for them all.

I had never imagined how lonely, frustrating, helpless, and pinned-down parenting could feel. How could I make room for how I was really feeling when it was this unattractive?

I didn't know it at the time, but this was the beginning of the eradication of the perfectionist in me. One of those tremendous blessings in disguise that at times feel like a sucker punch to the solar plexus. In other moments, they feel like a softening, a falling away of something diseased and dried up. Guess it depends on the day.

This experience of motherhood was working on me, kneading and shaping me into something previously unknown. I was given no choice, no alternative, no escape hatch. It was an experience of true immersion.

When something is working on us in this way, it is subtle yet steely strong. I could not see the effects at the time. All I could perceive was a gradual softening, becoming less stiff and contracted, better able to undulate with the flow of life. Snake was there with me too, reminding me to shed my expectations and assumptions. And in her healing form, she encouraged me to slough off old skins of regret and sadness, finding fresh layers of forgiveness underneath.

The truth is that this softening process carries on in me today, unfurling in supple, stretchy, living skin. Admittedly, there are still plenty of times I catch myself in restriction or attempts to harden as life continues to provide a steady stream of ongoing practice. I have had plenty of opportunities to say and do the wrong things, to feel the burn of shame, anger, or guilt. To rest in my bed at the end of a hard day and to sit quietly with the load of my feelings.

These are times when I engage in what I call *opposite prayers*. These intentions push against the easy, the bright, the accepted. Here are a few.

May I have the courage to feel this terrible, alone, and broken.

May I rest in the shadows for a while without flinching.

May I catch and stop my attempts at turning my real feelings into something more beautiful.

May I be brave enough to stay present with this oppressive weight, this slime of dread.

May I resist the tremendous urge to zone out, shift gears, leave, or bypass.

May I feel the nauseous squirming in my guts as a sign that I am a real, inhaling and exhaling human being.

May I not batten down the hatches of life so tightly that I think I will be impervious to life's waves, pretending I can outsmart suffering.

May my body follow the ups and down, the rise and fall of the ship, the weather sometimes flat and peaceful and at other times, invigorating, terrifying, lifegiving.

May I let the wind whip me and the sea spray drench me, feeling present with the fear and the spark.

In my experience it has only been in the incredibly unkempt panoramas of messy loving and crying, the irrational, uncontainable mayhem of parenting that the tightly raveled parts of me are reminded to release. And with regularity, my self-devotion is tested: Can I still love myself when it gets this unpredictable and uncomfortable?

Once you learn to return to self-love, failure becomes a little less terrifying. You are able to walk a little farther, dream a little bigger, and expand your heart a little further. You are able to risk the tightrope when there is always a soft cushion waiting for you, a velvety trampoline landing of unconditional acceptance.

Invoking the rebellious energy of the Space Dancer again, reflect on the idea of opposite prayers. Taking out your journal, write on the question/topic:

- *What methods may you sometimes use to bypass your uglier emotions for something more pretty or easy to swallow? What are the ways that you think you can outsmart your own suffering?*

- *What kinds of opposite prayers might you write for yourself?*

Every Damn Bump in the Road

Have you noticed how many times now I have used the "F" word? Yes, I have purposely chosen to use the word *failure* because I think we, as a human collective, need a shock to the system, a clap near the face.

I deeply believe in the magic and impact of word choice and the powerful symbolic codes words unlock for us. Look up *failure* in the dictionary and you will find that it is synonymous with "lack of success, collapse, deficiency, malfunction, loss, missteps and downfall."[9] Why would we want to associate ourselves with such a loaded, unpleasant word? Well, for sheer shock value, so we can shake the perfectionist by the shoulders and stare deep into her eyes and tell her she is making herself sick with the poison of extreme expectation.

We are only beginning to understand the deep roots of failure-aversion within our culture. Perfectionism is a persuasive and prevalent disease, sickening us into thinking that we will somehow be able to remain eternally mistake-free. It tricks us into thinking it will vaccinate us from all possible criticism in life.

Our inner perfectionist detests mess, chaos, unpredictability, or feeling out of control. We dress her, crown her, and make a pathway for her to sit upon her gilded pedestal. We might brag about her in job interviews: "I'm too much of a perfectionist" or "I care too much." ("I'm so dedicated, hardworking, and self-deprecating, oh my.") We cherish her ability to waste hours obsessing over the smallest of tasks, so that everything turns out "just right." With a whip in one hand and a leash in the other, she tightens that choker around our necks, expecting nothing less than the "very best" in every last thing that we do.

Somehow, she is able to let everyone else off the hook except herself.

This is because the inner perfectionist lives off a very special kind of fuel: fear of rejection. She thinks: *If I just keep working* (pant, pant) *as hard as a I possibly can* (pant, pant), *crushing all creative variability and flow in the process, I will* (wait for it . . .) *NEVER FAIL. I will never be criticized, I will never be unloved, I will never disappoint, I will never be left out, and more importantly, I will never be hurt.* In order to avoid this pain, she ratchets up the internal pressure. It is all she has control over, in a very out-of-control world.

Our inner perfectionist often chooses between two different modes of action: rumination or avoidance. When we ruminate, our inner analyzer gets put on high gear, spending way too long solving problems or dealing with the minutiae of life. This leads to a very fixed, tight, and constrained way of interacting with the world. We wear ourselves out without getting much done.

We run and run on the treadmill of our minds and never come to a resolution.

Most women are experts at falling into the prison of paralysis that ensues from constant analyzing. Once the trap has been set, we just keep on riding our mental loop for minutes, hours, and sometimes days. This is why I call this persona the Inner Ruminator: She is like a cow chewing her cud, grinding it down to a pulp, completely exhausting herself in the process.

Humans think we are the big-brained ones, but animals have a lot to teach here about being able to let go. Think about a cheetah stalking its prey: It spots an antelope, it's ready to bolt, and . . . off it goes. Poor little antelope, it zigs this way, then that way, every taut muscle in its body focused on escape. The cheetah is gaining, it goes in for one last pounce, and—the antelope turns just in time to escape its grasp. It bounds away, delirious and bone-tired.

Now, here's the important part. What does the antelope do right after it escapes? Does it take a couple of hours to rework the scene in its head, replaying how it could have turned here or jumped over there? No. Instead the antelope physically, vigorously shakes its body out, like it is shaking the trauma out of its tissues. And then it moves on.

Our large human brains really do come in handy a lot. We are capable of all sorts of dynamic understanding, communication, and logic. But the truth of the matter is that sometimes these big brains of ours get us into a whole bunch of trouble. Instead of living in the present, all that extra thinking keeps us stuck in the past. We waste a huge amount of time and energy replaying and reworking a certain event, interaction, or even a single word.

Another presentation of intense perfectionism is mega-procrastination, which is one more version of paralysis. Moving in circles, we get so wrapped up in making every little eensy-teensy thing just right that we get frozen before we can actually manifest or have an impact. We stop before we even start. This can be like stepping into concrete and not being able to go anywhere, too afraid to proceed out of the fear of not doing it right. Where is a sledgehammer when you need one?

Just talking about it, you can feel the perfectionist's internal pressure. I have a palpable sense of a pressure cooker with the lid on tight, steam bellowing out of any small cracks it can find. No matter what she does, the perfectionist believes that there is always an ample supply of doing better. Trying harder.

All of this self-induced pressure takes a toll. As a culture, we are only just beginning to understand the true mental, emotional, physical, and spiritual tolls perfectionism is taking on us. There is a slow-growing volume, voices being raised in protest that it deeply injures us. In the last decade, we have learned that perfectionists are more prone to anxiety, depression, self-harm, social anxieties, addictions, eating disorders, insomnia, hoarding, suicide, and overall burnout.[10]

Perfectionists feel every damn bump in the road with intensity, every faulty interaction or slight misstep. With their stress super-sensors switched on, operating like special little antennae, their systems get jarred by any unpredictable movement. In its most extreme version, women turn on themselves, engaging in mental (or even physical) cutting behaviors, knives slashing inside and out, punishing themselves for not living up to their own standards.

For too long, we have been glorifying perfectionism without studying its shadow side. It is high time we get deeply curious about this self-deprecating version of it because it is an enemy of the worst kind. It turns us against ourselves when we are meant to be our biggest allies.

It perpetuates a relentless feeling of not-enoughness.

It holds the censorship of joy and the repression of ease.

It crushes curiosity, wonder, and possibility right under its feet.

Do I think my perfectionistic tendencies have served me well? I can put my finger on the edge of something useful and admirable, but it is not the perfectionism. It is tenacity, hard work, an earnest desire to be fully engaged in my life with a deep sense of purpose.

My bones and heart speak of rebellion: I am done with all of this striving, trying to make myself into an unattainable work of art. I am so very tired of attempting to become some straight-A getting, metal sculpture of sorts. Taken too far, perfectionism causes us to forsake our very humanness, to turn away from life, or even worse, never to enter it. To be "perfect" implies that something is "complete, correct or flawless." But instead of making me feel more whole, my bouts with perfectionism have only made me feel more anxious, small, and fractured.

Sweet Pea Blossoms in a Jar

With all of this pressure to be perfect, my internal view finder was set on the relentless pursuit of outside rewards and outcomes, versus the inner work of genuine self-love. Perfectionism took a knife to the cords of confidence and self-trust within me, more and more threads fraying and severed with every passing of its blade.

I am using the past tense here, even though I still catch the perfectionist in me clawing to the surface every now and again. In times of overwhelm, the balances can get weighted in a certain direction and I start to orient from her push instead of from joy.

Sometimes it takes me a moment to notice her jab at my back with some invisible poker, trying to force me forward. But I notice her more easily now. She used to rule, crown and all, imperiously unchallenged. I don't respect her anymore, and that has drained the power out of her.

I no longer bow at her feet, but instead I search for the grace of imperfection all around me. I see:

The tearing, peeled-back edges of my journal.

The silent, small chip at the lip of my mug.

The rubbed patch of thinned and loved material on the couch.

The wind-caressed, slightly misaligned rope of prayer flags on my deck.

The mismatched gathering of highway-picked sweet pea blossoms in an old glass jar.

The cookies out of the oven, misshapen and lumpy, and still delicious.

The truth is that nothing in life should be too pretty.

The Japanese art of wabi-sabi is based in this very idea of imperfection and transience. Richard Powell, author of *Wabi Sabi*

Simple, describes how "Wabi-sabi nurtures all that is authentic by acknowledging three simple realities:

"nothing lasts,

"nothing is finished,

"and nothing is perfect."[11]

Even the term *wabi-sabi* feigns elusiveness and does not translate very easily. Author of *The Wabi-Sabi House,* Robyn Griggs Lawrence attempts with this description: "Wabi-sabi is the marriage of the Japanese *wabi,* meaning humble, and *sabi,* which connotes beauty in the natural progression of time."[12] She goes on to explain that "Pared down to its barest essence, wabi-sabi is the Japanese art of finding beauty in imperfection and profundity in nature, of accepting the natural cycle of growth, decay, and death."[13]

Over time I have come to search out and see wabi-sabi everywhere around me. This rich tradition provides an alternative perspective to the sleek, glossy, corporate style of beauty that has become the standard within western society. It is the opposite of the buy, buy, buy brainwashing that is constantly being pushed upon us. The philosophy of wabi-sabi questions our packrat existence and all the ways we continue to fill our burrows with the sparkle and shine of more stuff. For it is all this newness—wrapped in slick plastic—that conspires to convince us of the worthiness and normality of perfection.

Training in this world view of perfection constantly sets up expectations that leave no room for gray area, paradox, ambiguity, or the unknown.

It lays a suffocating layer of plastic over the possible.

I wish this plastic were entirely metaphorical, but sadly, we are literally, physically drowning in it: the micro-beads, sandwich baggies, food wrappings, shampoo containers, summer kiddie pools, pink alarm clocks, and airplane wings are seeping into us while also sinking into the oceans and soil. Plastics are being found in alarming levels in children's bodies and they are erupting out of the guts of almost all marine wildlife.[14] We are allowing this plastic perfection model to sink into the marrow of us physically and mentally. We are programmed into its filters of beauty: bleaching the teeth and hair, stretching the skin tightly, pulling, smoothing, hiding, coloring, with the unwritten expectation that we will be new forever.

But wabi-sabi reminds us of our transient, dust bodies returning to the Earth and of using natural materials, not synthetics. It encourages bicycle rust, weathering loveseats, fraying threads, hair-line cracks, and those stacked layers of forehead wrinkles. It is not in the sloppy, the cluttered, the disheveled, or the dirty, but in the simplicity of moss between cobblestone spaces, wandering orange poppies growing by the side of the road, the oxidation of silver bowls tucked in cupboards, and the mess of autumn leaves blown about your feet.

This art of imperfection takes what we think we should be, and it asks us to look deeper. And in this honest inquiry it wants us to find life infinitely more interesting. There is undeclared beauty all around us, but so often it is in the places that we least expect it or the places we still long to perfect. We might look for the very fullest moment of the moon's expansion—but what about when it hangs from the sky not quite full, imperfect as a pale apple with the slightest shaving along its flesh?

The philosophy of wabi-sabi asks us to be satisfied with what is in front of us. It lets us compassionately lighten up our expectations of ourselves and our world. It is freeing to make do with less. Instead of drifting through an endless desert of want, it sits us down into a nest of settledness, allowing a sense of enoughness to deposit into our own bones.

The gentleness of wabi-sabi may feel counterintuitive to confidence, but there is something earnest and hearty here if we really look. This is the confidence of humility, the confidence of modesty, the confidence of quiet, the confidence of deep observation. Exploring these qualities allows us to perceive that sometimes gentleness is its own form of strength.

Once again, we can challenge any false ideas that may try and convince us that confidence has to look like some smooth, pushy front. This is a more enduring self-devotion, the kind that knows that sitting as cargo within the fragile boat that carries us from birth to death, is the flawed or injured aspects of ourselves. A tremendous relaxation can move through us when we learn to navigate with, instead of against these gifts of imperfection.

Calling on the creative curiosity of the Artist-Visionary, explore the philosophy of wabi-sabi. With your journal ready:

- *Make a simple practice out of imperfection hunting. Wherever you are sitting right now, look around and jot down all of the things you see that are gloriously imperfect. How can you also allow yourself in be held in this view of natural imperfection?*

- *Even if you do not consider yourself a perfectionist, inquire if there are ways that you still long to control things in your life? How does using the viewpoint of wabi-sabi allow you to feel more satisfied with what is in front of you?*

The Fear-Trying Muscle

Coming to see, even encourage, the elegance of the simple, the well-loved, the awkward, the asymmetrical, the old, we can loosen the grasp we hold around ourselves. We can share the softness we have towards the imperfections all around us and include ourselves in this great loving circle. For there is unappreciated liberation in all of these shunned deficiencies.

Freeing yourself from the pressures of perfection opens the door to all sorts of new perspectives: the possibility of taking more risks, retraining ourselves about how we think about failure, and better seeing the ways we are constantly trying to block ourselves from criticism.

What so often holds women back is not our actual ability to act, compete, or perform, it's the choice we make when we decide not to try to reach for anything at all. It's the inertia that is the killer.

Remember, confidence builds in the doing, in the action, in the graduated steps forward. Confidence lives and breathes in the conclusion of your story, but you might not necessarily find it in the lines of the introduction. It might be fear instead that runs itself through those early pages.

Know that fear is protective, it alerts you to danger and it tries to sniff out hurt. Let fear speak to you, get interested in its voice instead of always cutting it off, rudely interrupting it with bad conversational manners. Let fear have its say.

But even after fear has gotten everything off of her chest, you may still feel scared to proceed. The more we can come into acceptance with this fact, the better we will be for it. It is the false belief that we should not feel fear that keeps us doubting ourselves and feeling like we are constantly doing something wrong.

So, start to exercise your fear-trying muscle. This is the action you will take while still feeling afraid. We must risk our way forward anyway. As Katty Kay and Claire Shipman write in *The Confidence Code*: "The confidence you get from mastery is contagious. It spreads. It doesn't even matter what you master: For a child it can be as simple as tying a shoe. What matters is that mastering one thing gives you the confidence to try something else."[15]

Sometimes confidence requires a gigantic leap and other times we have the opportunity to take baby steps in developing a new skill. Nansook Park, a psychologist at the University of Michigan who is an expert on optimism, talks about creating opportunities for graduated risk exposure, particularly as a way to build confidence in children. "They should be introduced to risk taking, but carefully. Don't just drop them in the middle of the lake. Teach them how to do things, then give them the opportunities, be there when they need guidance. When they succeed, celebrate together, and talk about what worked. And if they fail, talk about what they did well, the action should be the emphasis, but also what they can learn, and how to make it better the next time."[16]

This approach can be applied to adult women, too. Trauma obviously is not the goal in any new learning. Most of us know we could be taking more risks, but the baby step idea allows us to dip our toes in the shallow end a little bit, just long enough to get comfortable with the water temperature.

This might look like submitting your artwork to your local library before trying for your own big gallery show. Baby steps. Or it might be signing up for some public speaking classes before you accept that new job doing tons of presentations. Baby steps. The point is you don't need to stretch yourself to your most extreme breaking point— just stretch. Do something. Take an action.

The starting point for it all—risk, failure, perseverance, and confidence—is what Stanford University psychology professor and researcher Carol Dweck, Ph.D., teaches in her *growth mindset* work. In a 2012 interview, she discussed how with a "fixed mindset students believe their basic abilities, their intelligence, their talents, are just fixed traits. But in a growth mindset, students understand that their talents and abilities can be developed through effort, good teaching, and persistence. They don't necessarily think everyone's the same or anyone can be Einstein, but they believe everyone can get smarter if they work at it."[17]

Dweck's research has also found that a growth mindset especially correlates with higher levels of confidence in adolescent girls.[18] I get goosebumps just imagining what the world would look like if all young women learned to enter their adult years cultivating a growth mindset.

For when we are perpetual learners there is room for curiosity and investigation, room to move and explore in our lives. It is a fixed mindset that makes us afraid of challenge, afraid of reaching out, or afraid of rejection. But with an attitude of continual learning, we understand that nothing is set in stone. Curiosity supports bravery and resilience when and if we fail. And when we do get a firm no, maybe we lick our wounds in the dark for a little while. When we are ready, we can start again. We know that it is only through repetition, even when our heart is still sore, that creates a strong mastery-confidence continuum.

Wanting to turn our conditioning around failure and rejection on its head, the Space Dancer asks us to reimagine everything you have been taught. Surrounding yourself with a hefty dose of compassion, journal on the following questions.

- *Reflect on how your early life experiences influenced your beliefs about mistake-making. Instead of becoming completely paralyzed in the fear of failure, is there a way you can make it less scary, to set up soft trampolines of forgiveness and flexibility for yourself?*

- *We easily create resumes and report cards full of proving our goodness and worth. But what if you unabashedly created a "failure resume," a mock resume derived from losses instead of wins. I was introduced to this idea in Rachel Simmons' book* Enough as She Is. *Write down all of the mistakes, goofs, or dead ends reached, and treat them like blessings, achievements, and lessons wisely gained. To do this exercise, first describe the "setback" and follow it up with the "lesson."*[19]

Your Delicious Good

The musky, leathery smell of the patriarchy still lingered heavily on the chairs and desks when I went to high school. Mine had been an all-boys school for 180-something years before I got there and only a few years had passed since girls had been allowed entry into this legion of male history. On arrival, I felt unwelcome and out of place, like a rat in an experiment of unexpected social upheaval.

As part of the coeducational revolution, a number of new female teachers were hired and along with them came a slew of never-before-taught courses. One of them being an entire class on the selected works of Virginia Woolf. I couldn't perceive at the time what an impact this course would have on me, but it was a turning point in my thinking. It was as if my own teenage wit and brokenness connected to that of Woolf's and I quickly found myself lapping up her books like a homeless kitten drinks up a fortuitously found bowl of warm milk.

Woolf's writing was at times dark and weighted, while at other times strange, spirited, and fierce. Her insights pierced something in me, some yawning question around my life as a woman and of what I would be capable. I felt her life to have been like a vast troubled ocean, millions of black fins rising to many different rhythms, an endless rolling shimmering with no pattern at all. But her storminess was not a deterrent to me; I found her darkness magnetic. Somehow in understanding her, I hoped I could understand something more fully within myself.

Woolf was outspoken in depicting the stark contrast between how women were idealized in the fiction of her day as compared to how they were treated in real life. She gravely resented the social conventions imposed on women to be good girls, good wives, and good citizens. In her writings, she expresses that she felt to fully uphold the quintessential, societally appropriate role of "good girl," was to put a tourniquet on her own soul.

Woolf was in an ongoing dialogue with her inner good girl and could feel how this sacrificed version of herself always ended up putting everyone else's wishes before her own. She describes meeting this good girl in her writing:

The shadow of her wings fell on my page . . . Had I not killed her she would have killed me.[20]

Thinking about her work still conjures important questions for me: What within you dies when you are not able to express your true self? What masks do you wear, to make yourself look overly confident, overly nice, and overly in-control?

Woolf homes in on the expectation of women to "sacrifice herself daily," to give of herself so fully that there is nothing left—no time, no creativity, no inner wishes, no personal needs, no energy. To live like women routinely did in her day must have been like becoming a beautiful dish cloth, wrung out so completely that it stands up, rigid and parched, all by itself.

What are the lessons that modern women can learn from all of this sacrifice? We are still pleasing, even now. Especially in this Instagram age, it is so easy to curate the life you show the world, to paint pretty pictures in soothing colors, and only display smiles and accomplishments. Now more than ever, women are unconsciously struggling to keep up with the "shoulds" and "coulds," the projections fed to them by the container of our culture.

Is there a good girl who lives inside you, the pleasing one? Is she always waiting for an acknowledgment, some praise to strengthen her delicate shell? Does she want to feel some recognition of her potential desirability? A confirmation of being liked? An admission of a job well done? We are perpetually passing off our power when we seek our worth through our external achievements instead of our own self-actualization.

There are so many ways that we freely give away this power. Women learn from a young age never to act too proud, too smart, or too loud. Often our training is in actually putting ourselves down so that others will feel less threatened. It becomes taboo to share your triumphs but easy to commiserate about being stressed, overwhelmed, or exhausted.

This pandemic of reining-in is learned in early adolescence and it lingers in our tissues long after that. There is a reigning in that happens in order to not stand out, offend, or create jealousy, unconsciously endeavoring to cover up our brilliance and muzzle our opinions. Having internalized society's preferences, we become some tamer version of ourselves, wild horse spirits broken and well harnessed. The smell of rich leather in the air, we allow the cold metal of the bit to push hard against our palates, bowing our heads to allow our bridles to be positioned. Just. Right.

Sometimes it feels to me like there is an army of sameness taking over our culture as we are marketed and sold personalities that wear the uniform of monotony. Somehow, we believe that we will be safer and never criticized if we don't stand out. But Caroline Miller, a psychologist who specializes in confidence and optimism, says a willingness to be different is critical to confidence. She writes: "It's more than just risk and failure, though those are essential, confidence comes from stepping out of your comfort zone and working towards goals that come from your *own* values and needs, goals that are not determined by society."[21]

In other words, orient from your inner manifesto, that part of you that has already written and memorized your core guiding principles.

Its truths blaze.

In order to hear it fully you may even have to train in the radical skill of not giving a fuck. Which will feel awkward and foreign because most women are just not raised for it. The raw reality is that criticism and rejection burn long and hard. It is a kind of pain that we generally avoid at all costs. Criticism has this way of sucking us into vortexes of worthlessness or seemingly infinite, exhausting ruminations. But similar to any other practice, we must train in cutting our entanglements with other people, train in taking our energy back, train in believing in our own value.

Working with the practice of equanimity is helpful in seeing the ways we are habituated to constantly like, dislike, accept or reject every last little thing that comes our way. We can choose not to cling to the bad or the good feedback, but to instead see it all as someone else's opinions and thoughts. A noisy static of sorts. As painter Georgia O'Keeffe once said, "I have already settled it for myself, so flattery and criticism go down the same drain and I am quite free."[22]

I wish to bury the liberating essence of this quote into all of the corners of doubt in me. Outside interference goes down the drain once we realize that we have no control over what other people are going to think or say. Sometimes there may be something we can learn from the criticism. Other times we must adamantly repel what is not ours to take on, refusing to become trashcans for their judgments, insecurities, or assumptions.

Freedom comes when we drop ego attachment and wondering, *Do they like my art, my work, or me* and make up our own damned minds. In a way this leads us to a final sacred initiation, a crossing over of the threshold into total self-loyalty.

This is to take the faith, respect, and devotion that you hold for all of the things or people you really love and apply that same force towards yourself. We get a lot of practice being faithful to everyone or everything else: our partner, our job, our friends. But now we must create a habit of loyalty towards ourselves: devoted to our feelings, devoted to our flaws, devoted to our strengths, devoted to our truths.

Coming full circle now, what is it that you return to in your mind or in your life with habitual pull? I am wondering how the initiations of your life have directly impacted your strongest, repetitive mental stories. What if these stories could move you closer to yourself instead of farther away?

Looking to our animal teachers for examples of returning, we can feel into the stubborn biological persistence of the emperor penguin, green sea turtle, or Pacific salmon traveling back to the lands of their birth. With the magnetic force of circular migration, it is time for you to return to the natal grounds of your feminine confidence. Each time you take leave from your self-doubts and self-criticism and circle back to your sovereignty, you are practicing returning this energy to yourself, no longer wasting all of your delicious good.

Working with the penetrating insights of the Inner Healer, journal on these last questions.

- *Out of all the patterns in this chapter—pleasing, perfectionism, fixed mindset, fear of failure, rejection, or criticism—what tendencies do you return to the most in your life and why?*

- *Instead of continually strengthening these old stories and patterns, it is time to sit firmly within a deep sense of inner loyalty. Connect with this quality as a felt sense in your body and tune in to it as often as you can remember. Maybe you have a sensation of warmth through your heart or a weightedness in your pelvis. What subtle physical clues bring you to this inner-knowing? Journal on any other activities, practices, or new stories that return you to yourself, over and over again.*

May you have the confidence to hang out in the dark of the unknown when you need to, letting a torch of curiosity, patience, and trust light your way.

May you voluntarily shed skins when you are growing or disintegrating, feeling it to be part of the process of your own smaller death and birth cycles.

May seeing all of the imperfections around you lighten your load, allowing you to sigh and settle further into your flaws with loving honesty.

May you constantly swim in opportunities to practice having a mistake-making, perfectionist-killing, growth-mindset-swelling, fear-stretching outlook in life.

More than anything, may you know your bravery, that all of this spirited willingness to be vulnerable and in trust is not for the faint of heart. May you know self-loyalty like a heat, vibrating off of you, leaving contrails of confidence wherever you go.

CHAPTER SIX

Anoint Yourself

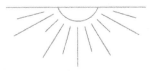

"Real love comes with a powerful recognition that we are fully alive and whole, despite our wounds or our fears or our loneliness. It is a state where we allow ourselves to be seen clearly by ourselves and by others, and in turn, we offer clear seeing to the world around us. It is a love that heals."[1]

—SHARON SALZBERG

The noises of everyday life disguised it for a very, very long time. Its first sound came as a soft, empty grumbling, followed by the cutting pang of hunger.

This pang began to insistently ache in me, a quiet protest of need. I came to the slow realization that I was *starving*. Starving by my own hand.

This was the creeping awareness that, despite all of my healing, evolving, and expanding, I was still offering myself nutrient-deficient scraps: discarded bits of easy compliments and obvious successes. Gathering the hand-me-downs of love when they happened to be available.

Heart Food

There is a deep hunger rumbling in the blackened hollows of many women. A drowsy awareness of how little they offer themselves still. Of how rarely they actually allow their spiritual bellies to be truly filled with all the beauty and grace of who they are.

Self-love is a root issue that too many of us keep dancing around, like a beautiful pool of water into which we briefly submerge our toes, but never quite get up the nerve to swan dive into.

Or if we do actually get in the "water" —temporarily embodying self-love for an evening or a weekend—we hop out again quickly, "drying off" too soon. Most of us don't spend enough time in the pool of self-love to become fully saturated by it, to let it soak past our skin into our cells and permanently transform our inner ways of knowing.

In order to understand the deepest recesses of feminine confidence, it is not enough to just dip ourselves in our own love periodically. We must immerse, becoming swimmers fully comfortable in the vast oceans of self- acceptance.

Self-love is a shapeshifter, fluidly capable of taking many different forms.

Love is an act of remembrance: traveling the old road rivers of deep soul knowledge.

Love is an act of softening: reminding our heart to stay as tender as a summer peach, juices running down our chins to get caught in the crevasses of fingers, lingering in stickiness.

Love is an act of bravery: having the courage to open the most delicate, baby-skin parts of ourselves to possible hurt or loss or betrayal. Love gives us the guts to embrace our own and others' repetitive shortcomings.

Love is an act of trust: like falling into the impartial warrior-like arms of a spiritual grandmother, who holds us with an energy of unconditional acceptance.

Love is an act of hard-core revolution: choosing hope and sanity, despite the sense of disintegration and suffering around us.

When we enter the expansive energy field of love, we find an ever-renewing intimacy with all things, including ourselves. Anointing ourselves with compassion is the labor of love we must return to over and over again until we feel confident that we can meet our challenges head on. In this way, self-compassion is the most direct pathway to self-confidence.

When we finally have the confidence to love ourselves absolutely, our default mode gets set on pulling ourselves in tighter, embracing ourselves more earnestly—and not just when things are easy or going our way. Vehement self-love knows that instead of shrinking it must embolden in strength, especially when we mess up or the winds of life push savagely against us.

Training ourselves to have this kind of reaction when we struggle to live up to our ideals lies in stark contrast to our rote response. In the past, we might have leapt at the chance to hand ourselves over to the inner critic. Addicted to the habit of self-criticism, we may think that by cutting ourselves down we are somehow making progress against our many flaws, which we have catalogued in detail. This pretend-bettering creates a routine of slashing and severing our self-trust, acting to reinforce and remind ourselves that we are nothing.

In fact, you may be hearing the voice of your inner critic right now, disparagingly taunting, *Is that it? Compassion leads to confidence? It can't be that basic!*

In the culture of the West, we tend to glaze over when someone tosses out words like *love* or *compassion*. We generally see these concepts as weak: airy-fairy and unrealistic. Love is for feeble-minded or naïve idealists. Compassion is thought to be a mushy, kumbaya thing that is attached to some false reality with a happy ending, ultimately unfit to stand up to the hard sensibility and aggressiveness of the real world.

The archetype of the Space Dancer reminds us that compassion actually contains many different faces and expressions. There is kitten fur-soft compassion and then there is a more intense, muscular version. One of my favorite stories that expresses this tough version of compassion is told by Lama Tsultrim Allione about a time she was having lunch with the Dalai Lama and some other Buddhist teachers, at the Spirit Rock Meditation Center in northern California. The conversation had turned to recent events of sexual misconduct within the western Buddhist community. One of the women in the group spoke up, describing how the members of her center were trying to work with one of the accused teachers with compassion, trying to understand the underlying reasons for his actions.

Surprising everyone in the room, the Dalai Lama pounded his fist on the table, exclaiming, 'Compassion is fine, but it has to stop! And those doing it should be exposed!'[2]

In that moment, the Dalai Lama exemplified a vision of fierce compassion: indisputably firm, clear, and piercing. The authoritative force behind his gesture was like a reverberation of thunder, a power yell erupting from deep in his fiery core: "NO, STOP, ENOUGH!"

This kind of compassion has bite. With its flashing eyes, blood-soaked fangs, eagle-sharp claws, it is the opposite of wishy-washiness. But it isn't aggression. It does not rule for ruling's sake or squeeze you with power for the delight of hurting you. It is a raw, undeniable force, embodied in the image of a threatened, charging mother bear, her mouth salivating, hot grunts releasing, moving with pure instinct.

Fierce compassion cuts, cuts, cuts away with the teeth of discernment, pulling fascia away from muscle, continually moving you closer to the bone of truth.

Understanding that there can be a ferociousness to compassion gives us insight into the fierce feminine. Discernment of its nature comes after finally accepting that we as women can embody so many moods, so many different weather patterns, so many seemingly contradictory qualities: both yin and yang, soft and hard, quiet listening and assertive space-taking, a yes and a no.

Receiving yourself fully is a subversive, rebellious act of self-compassion. The truth is that it takes greater strength to choose to accept yourself, stretch marks, stains, flaws, and more, than to keep punishing yourself for your supposed imperfections.

We must finally come to see that we can't unrestrictedly give to others what we don't yet know how to give to ourselves. But why do our arms rest wide open for others and hang limply by our sides when it comes time to embrace ourselves?

Deep cultural, familial, or religious persuasions initiated long ago have indoctrinated generations of women into ideas around selflessness and unbalanced giving. This may have been how we learned to be worthy of love: by taking care of other people. On some level, we may always feel the overlord of guilt waiting for us, expecting us to hand over a piece of ourselves. The voice of guilt is quick to remind us that self-love and -compassion are indulgent and selfish, or maybe even narcissistic.

Now don't get me wrong, there is absolute and unequivocal beauty in giving to others. But so many women have taken this heartfelt, compassionate idea and twisted it into something sickly. When we hide behind our giving to others, too scared to feel like we ourselves are worthy of receiving, we end up hungry, depleted, and hollow.

The source of true kindness first begins within to then be shared outwards. We must learn to feed ourselves well in order to confidently give *and* receive. When our reserves are full and overflowing, when we are soaked and sopping with self-love, then giving has a naturalness, becoming healthy and less complicated.

Working out our doubts and hesitations about self-love once and for all is absolutely necessary to fully embody feminine confidence. We have to do love to do confidence. When we return to love, steady in our cores, confidence is able to radiate from a sense of inner abundance and sufficiency, dare I say it, *happiness* even.

Inspirational speaker Danielle LaPorte offers us this gem on self-love: "My journey to love myself can be summed up in one word: *softer.* The closer I am to my essence, the softer I become, I'm still fierce, even fiercer in some ways, but I can be on my own edge without becoming edgy. More fluid, less angular."[3]

I love this intersection of fierce and soft, edge without edginess, returning to the fluid, ocean waters of love within us.

Let me offer you meals of self-love now, heart food for the places in you that may be quietly starving. When we have retrained our default mode in self-love and compassion, when we have worked it out within our internal landscape, our feminine confidence easily shines into our external world. We must stop cutting ourselves off from love. Instead, let us bring the heart food of self-love close and palatable, never allowing ourselves to go so hungry again.

Fundamental, Unconditional, Unshakeable

The truth is that the love in us is as basic as the moon in orbit or the gravity that keeps us from floating towards the vacuum of space. It is as fundamental as the Earth beneath our feet and the rawness of our naked bodies. It is as basic as the sun rising in the East and setting in the West.

So far, these facts haven't changed on us. We do not question their consistency or realness. And the same is true of our basic nature. From this point of view, we have everything we need, so that we don't feel like we are constantly at arm's length from the world. We have been equipped with an inherent worth that is unshakeable.

In the Shambhala Buddhist tradition, the experience of unconditional worthiness is called *basic goodness.* The word *good* in this context does not mean *better than,* as in some dominating sense. *Good* does not hold up in direct comparison to *bad* because there is nothing bad when we are talking about human nature. Instead, *good* signifies something complete, untouched, and totally worthy of existence.

The idea of basic goodness can be very difficult to swallow deep inside us when we have so much training in our sins, in our wickedness, in our need to confess, repent, be cleansed. Western culture has inherited a viewpoint that human beings are intrinsically imperfect, flawed, and aggressive, and this idea has spread throughout human history and across most religions and cultures. Pema Chödrön calls this the view of *basic badness,* working to unconsciously shape the foundation of our hearts and minds.

After so much powerful conditioning we are pretty attached to the view of basic badness, and a vague sense of fragile unlovability may always be waiting for us. We are convinced of the need to constantly seek outside of ourselves for some flimsy reassurance and confirmation of our worth and desirability. This puts us in the precarious role of a passive recipient of love, always waiting, hoping, allowing ourselves only the little bits and scraps of whatever happens to come along.

Stories and training from our past may continually convince us that we must prove our good. From this viewpoint, our value lies in what we do, rather than in who we are. Accordingly, we must always be doing, doing, doing in order to prove our real worth. And many of us have fully tested this theory, working ourselves to some death, fingers toiling, dry bones clicking away like knitting needles.

Just because we are all born ready to love and be loved does not mean that all of us live this way. I promise you nothing that saccharine sweet. The human experience is rife with complex layers of betrayal, trauma, heartbreak, and all sorts of other pain that often convince us of brokenness, within ourselves, others, even the world at large. Just because our essential nature is love does not mean that a thick cloud of suffering and confusion doesn't often hang over us, obscuring our ability to find any shred of goodness in each other.

It seems like common sense that if at least some of our species did not possess the potential for tenderness and altruism in our chromosomes, we would have all killed each other off long ago. And often from our modern news coverage, we are brainwashed into feeling like this is actually happening. Yet there are acts of tremendous altruism, generosity, and care happening every day in the smallest and largest of ways, sometimes behind closed doors, and other times right in front of us.

We might encounter clear acts of kindness, and yet somehow, their beauty rolls off of us like water off a duck's feathers, never really penetrating deeply into our consciousness. How would our global mindset be altered if we had news coverage on all the simple, loving acts that happen every day? How would it feel to go through life invested in the integrity of others?

So many of us are rooting for goodness and sanity. At this very moment, there are:

- Tibetan monks somewhere, chanting for the cessation of the suffering of all beings.
- Nuns in the Alps holding a ceaseless vigil, praying for all of God's children.
- Numerous kundalini yoga classes using voice and body to tune into the divine flow, to bow to the ultimate teacher within.
- Holy places all over the world that are giving human beings a chance to connect to something sacred, no matter what religious coat it wears.
- Thousands upon thousands of people in meditation and prayer, opening their hearts to shine their lights throughout the world.

- Innumerable acts of beauty, kindness, and care that people are gifting to others, such as holding the hands of the dying, the wounded, and the scared.
- Countless children being kissed and hugged by their loving parents, giving them the love, attention, and presence that they need to feel cared for.

The good news is that no matter what kind of people we encounter in life or how we are treated, our unconditional worthiness cannot be taken away from us. It is not based on the grandness of what we achieve or how perfectly we make house or the opinions of our colleagues and employers.

It is not grading you.

The gem of worthiness inside you just keeps on glowing, steady and strong, unimpacted by the external details of your life. This worthiness is oblivious to your biggest flaws, unconscious blunders, and gut-wrenching failures. And, of course, it goes without saying that all humans possess worthiness innately, regardless of sexuality, gender, race, or class. Thus, it binds us together and lets us breathe in sync.

In his book *The Age of Empathy*, biologist Frans de Waal details how both animals and humans have an innate sensitivity that enables them to read each other's faces and bodies as a way to understand emotions.[4] By studying the social behaviors of many different kinds of animals, de Waal has documented how animals (and humans) are programmed to reach out. He has found that chimpanzees try to help a wounded mate, elephants provide reassuring "rumbles" to upset young ones, and dolphins support sick companions near the water's surface to prevent them from drowning. Whales have been known to protect and hide seals (and even a human) under their fins, away from sharks and other predators.[5] Despite presiding ideas that humans are violent and aggressive, de Waal presents an argument that there are biological roots to human kindness.[6]

This is to remember the basic goodness of everything, knowing that there is no bad chipmunk, no bad willow tree, no bad hawk, no bad wind, no bad cloud—and no bad human. It is somehow easier to feel this direct inheritance through the model of the living world. I think of the essential nature of that barred owl from earlier pages as unwavering and unquestionable as you dear reader, sitting here taking in this book.

Yes, there is room for us humans in this too. There is no bad me and there is no bad you. This moment is complete just as it is and so are you. You were born okay the first time and, in this way, your true nature cannot be touched by the worst of life.

Your Inner Healer understands that you were created worthy of love. You don't even have to do anything exceptional to prove it. You are love. Let her guide you now as you take some time to write on these questions:

- *Free write about the basic goodness and naturally confident manner of everything around you. Reflect on how you are not separate from all of life—this goodness is your direct inheritance too.*

- *If it feels challenging to connect with your basic goodness, start with baby steps. Honor your basic human desire to be happy, healthy, and safe. Start that small. And then connect with this basic human desire in others, that they too long to know love, to be free from hunger, loneliness, or pain. Write about these baby steps of basic goodness.*

- *Believing in the goodness of our essential nature and our worthiness of receiving love, flex the muscles of love instead of the muscles of self-sabotage. Self-love is an ever-unfolding process, a routine, a practice, a habit that you train yourself towards over and over again. Let this love for yourself be something you can return to, steely strong arms you know you can rely on and come home to. These arms are always available for you no matter how lost you might feel or how many fumbles you might make. Write on what these arms feel like to you.*

I Am Another You

Let yourself know your own essential worthiness and let yourself see this same worthiness in others—in your parents, in your coworkers, in your children, and in your most annoying neighbor. Yes, despite their flaws they are deserving of love. See through to their inner vulnerabilities, best intentions, shortfalls, and perpetual dilemmas. Know that even when other people's behavior doesn't always make sense to you, they are doing their best in their own way.

Loving ourselves with compassion makes it easier to extend that same kind of compassion towards others. What if this compassionate love itself could be reclaimed as a larger public ethic? This is the question proposed by civil rights activist and lawyer Valarie Kaur, the creator of the Revolutionary Love Project. Her social justice movement envisions a planet where love is a wellspring for social change and a force of good against racism, nationalism, and hate. The Revolutionary Love Project is rooted in a three-part declaration: "We are claiming our love for the other, especially those in harm's way, claiming our love for our opponents, even when they hurt us, and claiming our love for ourselves, the foundation on which it all rests."[7]

Kaur's movement to make our legal system more equitable is based in the wisdom that those that hurt others are themselves threatened, afraid, wounded, and cut off from love, and we need to see past their hate and into their fear. She teaches that "when we reclaim love through a feminist lens, then love is a form of sweet labor. Fierce. Bloody. Imperfect. Life giving. A choice we make over and over again."[8] I deeply respect her insight that the ethic of love is what is needed to birth a new era.

This approach is to know love for the subversive power it contains. Love acts as a bridge that lets us traverse the moats of separation inhabited by the snapping alligators of assumption. Working with the idea of no-separation is a healing path to mend some of the deepest rifts within our society.

For many Indigenous cultures around the world, reciprocity is the most foundational of all principles. In the ethnolinguistic Mayan culture of Central America, the phrase *In lak'ech* basically means "I am another you," and *ala k'in* means "You are another me." So, it is custom to greet someone, *"In lak'ech ala k'in,"* which essentially means "I am you and you are me."[9] The Mayans understand the importance of mutual kinship and the oneness of everything.

Imagine what the rest of the world would look like if we modeled our behavior after the Maya and truly searched to see ourselves in others. Could we remember that, on some cross-cultural, foundational level as human beings, people of every walk of life and background are not that dissimilar? We all want to laugh, to eat, to drink, to love, to be surrounded by family and friends, to know basic rights and comforts.

When we work with an attitude of availability towards others, we remain open, without automatically cutting others down out of our own fear or insecurity.

When we abstain from criticism or ill will against another person, we also are agreeing subliminally to banish that same kind of judgment and hostility towards ourselves.

When we appreciate the tremendous, spectacular brilliance and talent in someone else, we also vow to see those things in ourselves.

When we recognize that others around us are doing their best, it means that we are also open to recognizing our own positive intentions and efforts.

Love is like a revolving door. Whatever we put out circles back to us. Around and around we go, giving and receiving in an exchange of energy and emotion during each interaction. This phenomenon begs the question: Are we ready to love ourselves with the same magnitude of intensity and heat that we love those whom we care about most?

Calling on the honest wisdom of your own Inner Healer, contemplate and write on the following questions:

- *Create a habit of regularly asking, "Where can I resource from love, instead of unconsciously protecting the demands of my frightened self?"*

- *What does the style of criticism that I use to judge or criticize others have to reflect about how I judge or criticize myself? How does it reflect my deeper wounds, insecurities, and fears?*

- *Valerie Kaur suggests you ask: "What would it take to bring the wellness I want in the world into my own home?"[10] Reflecting on that question you might consider: What changes would need to occur in your life to have it mirror the kind of world you want to live in? How does loving yourself in this way open you up to teaching and modeling to others a new way of using love in the world?*

Becoming an Ocean

Great love holds the hand of great forgiveness. They are Gemini twins who wander around attached, seemingly incomplete without feeling the other walking right there beside them.

A supernova of love blasts open when we consciously let the work of forgiveness out. This is not forgiveness from a letting-go or being-done-with-it perspective. It is not a forced ceasefire of resentment or hatred—although these things may come about as positive side effects over time.

When you know yourself in another being, once again you clean up your view of separation. You can see beyond the limits of your brain and eyeballs and peer into the world of another to witness his or her own fragile humanness.

This is a style of forgiveness that softens betrayal when someone you trusted fails you. That someone could be your mother, your father, a teacher, a partner, or society at large. You can start to breathe from their lungs and see through their eyes and begin to know their fears, insecurities, regrets, deep programming, and bruises from a life lived as a flawed, complicated, often well-meaning human being.

It is tiring to constantly check our wounds and keep our bandages clean. It is exhausting to keep our old stories fresh, to pretend like they are still interesting and worthy of repeating. Forgiveness has a wide, warm lap to hold us in wholeness, to gently take the burden from our hands.

Forgiveness may ask us to become an ocean, growing bigger with every pulsation of our hearts. As an ocean, cups of burning salt can be added to our immense stocks of water but our capacity for compassion swells in these vast waters. As we expand ourselves outwards in presence and strength, there is a diluting of our limiting stories. The water molecules within the amniotic fluid of these inner seas holds a message of cosmic consciousness: "Whatever has happened to you in your life, it cannot change who you are on the deepest level."

This is a forgiveness that has soft, warm waves on which to rock the grief in us. Let these boundless waters wash you clean, from the smallest slights of childhood to your still-fresh adult wounds. More than anything, make room for yourself in these glorious waters; enjoy the cathartic cleanse of including yourself in the forgiving.

Forgive yourself for all of the ways you have held yourself back, all the ways you crucified yourself. All the heart-penetrating criticisms, the tragic self-talk, the inner barbed wires that have kept you tight, stunted, and trained in smallness.

You may have been the one who decided you were not good enough.

At some point, you may have failed to fight for your own life.

When we really touch into these regrets, we meet its emotional depth and the potential for healing through grief. We behold a cavernous sadness for not having been our biggest ally all along. For not holding ourselves, caring for ourselves, listening to ourselves, upholding our needs above everything else. All the years wasted in doubting that we had something valuable to share.

Like a mother grieving the loss of her child, in doing the work of examining our shadow remorse, we may feel into the regrets of the unnourished self. This part of us wants to be acknowledged in order to be reintegrated and made whole again. Acknowledging our sadness becomes its own sacred anointing.

Animal teachers show us how to grieve. Chimpanzee mothers refuse to put down their dead babies.[11] Crows cry and cry for the breaking of the bond with their life partners.[12] And elephant herds ceremoniously touch the bones of a found elephant carcass, a natural act of reverence.[13]

Reading through NPR one day, I was transfixed by the story of Tahlequah, a mother orca whose baby had died.[14] Tahlequah's calf was born alive and actually swam by her side for about thirty minutes before it perished. Her story lodged itself in my heart and later that day I imagined in my journal what it had been like for Tahlequah's calf.

How utterly peaceful to be rocked this way. To grow and be nurtured in this watery home of a womb. To share bodies and to have the sounds of each other's heart beats reverberate off one another. To rely on each other's presence so intimately for an entire seventeen months.

After her baby passed, Tahlequah gathered its body and carried it with her. Now it is not uncommon for orcas to swim with the carcass of a baby for a day or two, but this was not enough for her. No, her tour of grief lasted seventeen days and a thousand miles as she divided the task of carrying her baby with other pod members, giving them a chance to share in the sadness.

Orcas are a matrilineal species, dependent on their mothers and grandmothers to lead their pods. For a while it was unclear if

Tahlequah would put the entire pod in danger by adding her own death to the abysmal statistics of orca fatalities, due to taking on the exhausting task of carrying this extra weight. But after seventeen days, she was complete somehow.

Who understands this mystery of when we are done grieving? I imagine the baby orca's well-loved body sinking gently to the ocean's floor, to be embraced by the cycle of living and dying, absorbed and decomposed in completion.

We have to wonder what Tahlequah was experiencing to make such a profound expression of mourning to the world. What would it be like to be underwater and hear her clicks and squeaks of heartache echoing through the depths?

Her act of anguish touched something submerged within me when I read about it. And her story made me wonder what would happen if we went on our own tours of grief, created our own rituals to mark the past. What would it look like to carry some younger part of ourselves, to gently cradle our hurts for a while?

What would it be like to acknowledge how painful it has been when we have not practiced self-compassion?

How might your life feel more complete by integrating these neglected parts back, kindly folding them into the mix of your healing and wellbeing?

On the last check I know of, Tahlequah was spotted with a new baby in the beginning of September 2020.[15] There is hope that beyond the grieving lies something yet undiscovered, that the push to live pulses in us all.

Invite in a sense of forgiveness towards yourself right now for all of the unconscious ways you reacted and lived according to the influences of your cultures and let your inner-critic rule. Now allow the Inner Healer to tend your heart, reflect on the idea of forgiveness for yourself and others in your journal.

- *What if you were to hold those younger/older parts of yourself that you may have denied, hurt, starved, or betrayed and finally acknowledge the times you did not fight for yourself? If you feel like you need to go on your own tour of grief, what would it look or be like?*

- *On some level you may believe that you can't forgive your biggest hurts, that you can't possibly let go of the wounds that have defined you and possibly written the lines of your life's story. For a little while, imagine yourself as an ocean and explore how it feels to soften these storylines, diluting them a bit, calming their charge, holding them with compassion.*

Explorations of Love Joy

Grounded within the unconditional worthiness of ourselves and others, now is our opportunity to remember self-love through three creative explorations. Self-love feeds the confidence and willingness we need for all creative risk-taking.

Let us begin with a couple of simple equations: Love = Joy and Joy = Love. If your heart needs baby steps to find its way to anoint yourself with love, start by looking at these states of being within the experience of your everyday, current reality. Look for opportunities to feel joy or love in the obvious location.

Right where you are.

Joy and love are not in hiding from you, in fact quite the opposite. They are right there, in front of your nose, all day long. It is the Love + Joy connection, the awkward beauty, the moldy decay, and the painfully mundane that lifts our spirits. All of the stuff that is right there in front of us that we are usually just too oblivious or busy to see.

As the Buddhist teacher Chögyam Trungpa Rinpoche says: "Our lives awaken through ordinary magic."[16] He was speaking to the everyday enchantment and ease of love and joy, always closer than we realize. We have a constant opportunity to interact passionately with the world around us and take joy in doing so.

What is physically right in front of me is Merlin, the wizard-like sequoia in my backyard. His great arms stretch wide to the sky, although there are many places where his branches have been trimmed, leaving layers of circular scars. Like a solemn totem pole, his circles resemble eyes looking out in all directions. Eyes belonging to the many animal spirits of the land: coyote, deer, raccoon, squirrel, bald eagle, spotted towhee, and banana slug.

Merlin is unmistakably the king of the land, upright and regal, his rusty-colored bark absorbing and shining even more intensely in the summer sunsets, radiating its own bonfire light. I regularly adorn him with stones, petals, and various other nature refuse, although he drops so many tree bits that everything which I devotedly lay down quickly vanishes.

Trees are slow-moving animals. Just because they seem stationary doesn't mean they aren't living, trembling wonders. Today we understand that trees are communicating and collaborating through an underground *mycorrhizal network,* which is a function of the symbiotic relationship between fungi and plants. But there is so much for us to further understand about how a forest acts as a single organism, exchanging chemical and bioelectric signals through their root systems.[17]

Like humans, trees are very social creatures and depend on each other for survival. We know they are vital to our ecosystem, but we mostly forget (or never knew) that we live in biological unity with these beings. Our breathing cycle exists in an exact opposite pattern from that of trees: We release carbon dioxide and they process this to, in turn, release oxygen as an offering of life. In turn, we have evolved biologically to mirror these plants, our lungs the holographic image of two living trees.

It is through the release of their aromatic, volatile oils that we are gifted with their ancient pranic intelligence, as well as their pharmacopeia of immunological genius. These respiratory tree oils contain antifungal, antibacterial, and antimicrobial medicine; having soaked up all the wisdom of their ancestral history, as well as all of the energy, sunlight, and moonlight in their environment.

Yes, I live in a constant state of dendrophilic reverence. But what lights you up so that you just can't stop talking about it?

What happens because you love? This is the perfect moment to get out your journal and start to free-write about your small joys.

- *What ways could you use joy as the precursor to love? How can you expand this love both inwards and outwards?*

- *What else happens because you love? Begin a casual list. For example, "Because I love":*

    ". . . microscopic miracles are given permission to unsnarl and explode into reality."

    ". . . the stars do their masterful ceremony every night, singing the song of the ancient ones."

    ". . . life force continues to flow through my veins, pinkening my skin, and shining light through my eyes."

    ". . . the seasons mature into each other, the rivers push, the mountains hum and the continual braid of life and death weave their way through everything."

Explorations of the Magical Child

I keep a picture of myself as a baby on my desk, along with a colorful array of pictures and poems of inspiration. No, it is not some form of self-idolization; rather, this old polaroid has a way of sustaining me. It reminds me of a simpler time when all I knew how to do was radiate love.

Apples for cheeks, pudgy and pink all over, in this snapshot I have a look of absolute elation and joy on my face. I sense a twinkle of trickster in my eyes. It is in this white baby romper with an elfin hood that I could do no wrong.

There were no self-doubts, no self-hatred, no shame.

I didn't yet know to question the validity of my existence. I was just hanging out as my miracle-self, pleased to be awake and alive. I was doing what I was born to do: let all the stars of the universe blaze out of my every little pore.

She is me and I am her.

I can feel that this bliss baby is still in me somewhere. Of course, I am very content with not being an actual drooling, helpless infant. (There are big benefits to talking and walking!) I will take the adult roller-coaster ride of living with radical engagement, thank you very much. But at the same time, I can sense that this unencumbered, innocent Buddha babe is still giggling her cute little behind off right now, inside of me. This is the young, yet very wise part of me that has no doubts about her essential nature.

Travel with me now, to the time of your birth. I want you to take a moment to feel all the joyful goodness that cradled you at that time. Feel into the unending nebula of love that embraced you, the people that acknowledged your wholeness and radiance.

The truth is that most of us hold a story about our births that is the opposite of this. Maybe in our story, our birth is filled with chaos, fear, or being unwanted. Maybe we were born into violence, illness, or a pit of loneliness. Or maybe we hold no story or knowledge at all; perhaps if we were adopted those details were deliberately hidden from view. Or we may have been passed down a birth story of apathy, taking it all in as mediocre.

Stay with me here. What if you allowed yourself to rewrite the story that you have? Instead of focusing on all the wrongs or absences, imagine how your story would change when written by the magical child. From the viewpoint of the magical child, you are loved, you are seen, and you know trust.

The magical child is not worrying about the future, she only knows the eternal present. She lives in deep time: time that unfolds at the pace of a decomposing tree. Time that remembers when oceans were deserts and desserts were oceans. Time like the evolution of species. Time like snow consciousness. Time like a hand reaching back through the hearts of our ancestors.

She knows every atom of her being as the Great Mystery. She sees her birth as tenderly fortunate. She does not question her place, her worthiness, or her ability to feel, share, and receive love. There is no hesitation in her knowing. Loving everything. That is why she is here.

Every child wants to be seen, really seen, all the way down to the depths of his or her sweet soul. Children want to be seen for their light and joy and they are magnetized by what feels most vibrant around them. They do not want to be seen through the lens of their culture's or parent's ideas, rules, restrictions, and stories about them. The soul has very different needs from the ego. The ego is the psychological structure that helps us interface between our inner and outer reality. But the soul has a life of its own, beyond the constraints of the "you should."

Connect with that soul child, that running free part of yourself that says "I'm alive, really alive within you!" I want you to envision beyond the constraints of your life. Let the love you stir up penetrate all the layers of your being.

Try this same exercise at home now. Start with reflecting on an old baby picture of yourself. Taking out your journal, begin to free-write on the name Magical Child. How does it feel to connect with the love, joy, and magic that you came in with, that is still bubbling within you? How easy or hard is it to access this part of yourself?

Explorations of the Divine Love Note

Imagine your own best friend is already living inside of you. Not the bitchy, overbearing kind, but the compassionate, faithful type. The let's-forget-the-small-talk and get-down into the darkest-messiest-sex-magic-death-atoms-faraway galaxies part-of-your-soul kind of friend.

Your best friend knows that you, like all of us, exist in a transient expression of sacredness. We each hold an ecological niche on this Earth. Just like the pattern of your fingerprints, no one is exactly like you, not even a twin. At the moment of your birth, the planets in the sky were arranged in a divine pattern, creating an energetic imprint on your consciousness. There may have been other babies born on the same day, even at the same minute, but none of them were born in that location to your mother. You are a rare entity, never to be created exactly the same again.

I don't mention this to boost your ego or to urge you into further attachment to the idea of being a separate self. This is not a place from which to build yourself up artificially or to think you are better than other beings. This is about recognizing the preciousness of your human birth and the extraordinary gift that has been given to you. There is an old story from the Pāli canon, a set of ancient sacred scriptures from the Theravada Buddhist tradition, in which the Buddha explains that a human birth is very rare. He says:

Suppose that this great earth was totally covered with water and a person was to toss a yoke with a single hole into the water. A wind from the West would push it East; a wind from the East would push it West; a wind from the North would push it South; a wind from the South would push it North. And suppose a blind sea turtle were there. It would come to the surface only once every hundred years. Now what do you suppose the chances would be that a blind turtle, coming once to the surface every hundred years, would stick his neck into the yoke with a single hole?[18]

This metaphor sums up the probability of you being born in human form. The possibility of you, exactly as you are now, is the same magical likeliness as a blind turtle sticking its head through that yoke, in all those great oceans, once every hundred years. Don't take this miracle for granted.

If you were to write a sacred love letter to yourself, what would you say? Would there be apologies, regrets, or tears of softening? Acceptance of flaws and mistakes, and an offering to keep learning? To know your crystalized scars and the places that still make you frozen? To look past the massive canyons of fear to the unknown frontiers of possibility? To be surprised by your tender resilience and lioness courage?

To know yourself as a wild bloom, fierce and fragile, enchanting and imperfect?

Okay, time to disrobe. As Natalie Goldberg says in *Writing Down the Bones,* "Go for the jugular" (she meant about writing of course, but I find myself repeating this line in times of doubt, regardless of the topic).[19] Here is my sacred love letter.

Dear Sorcerer of Beauty,

I love you, dear Phoenix, in all the many ways you have risen from the ashes, stronger and more passionate than ever to live.

I love your daring heart and how you continue to peel back the layers, the remnants and paper-thin wisps of who you used to be.

I love your tenacity for truth and your willingness to be rolled over, tumbled, worn away, ever softening into a sacred trust.

I love your tremendous capacity to give of yourself, to share, to let your heart be a thousand-pointed star.

I admire your willingness to be born again into failure and to say farewell to the quickly dissolving Queen of Perfect.

I admire your persistence to stick with what is currently arising, radiant, confused, radiant, frustrated, radiant, alone, radiant, stuck, radiant, enough.

I admire your desire to break the ancestral ties that bind, the unhealthy imprints and unwanted stories.

I admire the vow you took to see love, feel love, be love, live love—for that is all we have.

May you always be present in your authentic self.

May you always feel your right to be here and take up space.

May you continue to align with your true responsibility, the ever-evolving journey of your soul.

Now it is your turn to write. What beautiful rhythm of words wants to pour forth, opening a stream of tenderness and self-compassion in you?

If you feel stuck, you can try to first do a free-write with the prompt: What does the wide-open heart of my inner best friend want to tell me about enoughness? See what words want to dot the page and then grow and develop your feelings from there.

This should not be a pep talk letter or a this-is-what-you-need-to-work-on letter. Quite the opposite. It is a letter infused with your basic worthiness, your deepening self-love, and the blessing of self-forgiveness.

Hatched by Your Own Warmth

Chew slowly. As if you are a rich, satiated woman.

We work hard to change our material circumstances, but without cultivating a sense of inner richness, a feeling of deep dissatisfaction always persists.

Our perpetual sense of needing more not only leads to a lot of unintended purchases, unintended snacking, and a variety of other unconscious behaviors, it also lies at the root of something much more profound. The idea that there is some deep bottomless pit within us that will never feel stocked, no matter how much we lovingly put in. That all our actions to feel meaningful are actually fueled by a deep fear of being insignificant.

If there is a solid sense of confidence and contentment inside, it breaks the cycle of always needing to put our suckers out, searching for more. This inner richness arises from a feeling of hearty completeness, saturating the center of every cell.

You have enough and you are enough.

I see this in you now . . .

Every day, may you be your own mother sitting on the egg of your original sacredness.

May you never need the incubator of your culture to know your own value. May you never rely on the heat of another to validate your inherent completeness.

May you be hatched by the warmth of your own love. To brush and braid your hair with the gentleness of a doting grandmother.

May you be hatched by the warmth of your own kindness. To touch your skin with the care of the most attentive lover.

May you be hatched by the warmth of your own compassion. To know the voice of your own calling as "dear one," "sweetheart," and "my love."

May you be hatched by the warmth of your own softness. To wrap yourself up in the sweater of forgiveness and have a nap from the endless inner grind.

May you be hatched by the warmth of your own gentleness. To place your hand on your heart, and to love and love and love until the rhythm of its uncontainable pulsing is an echo of resounding strength vibrating out of every pore.

May you crack your shell, free into this world, inherently knowing the song that is only yours to sing, a bird taken flight on the currents of her own power and truth.

CHAPTER SEVEN

Waters of Restoration

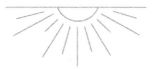

"True confidence—divine confidence—comes from the deep knowing that we are spiritual beings, whole beings, human beings who are mysteriously and magnificently part of the One, and not separate at all. . . . The courageous warrior within you—the one who has fought the gravitational pull of shame, hurt, hopelessness and despair—is the keeper of your divine confidence. And she will help you claim your most holy reason for being."[1]

—DEBBIE FORD

Slick and amphibian, I became a creature of currents and repetition while doing laps. There is something that changes inside of you when you submerge yourself this way, the rhythm of your inhale, hold, followed by your exhale, hold. Taking one length of the pool at a time because there is no other way. The sheer immensity of it, the number of laps expected of you, counting in twos through ten, and then sixty and beyond. And then my mind would change my counting strategy again, maybe moving into fives, as a way to pass the time, to stay sane.

Work First, Spirit Later

I swam through it all.

Through exhaustion and ambition and leg cramps. Through apathy and the vice of my period and earaches. Complete boredom and exercise-induced bliss. When I felt like I could go no further, I would ask, "What if I go further?"

These laps were my introduction to meditation, teaching me to rest in the chanting of my breathing, the vague echoes of thoughts coming and going underwater. Perhaps this dreamy landscape aided in me feeling the very temporary, aqueous quality of my mind. That it could all dissolve given the chance—even the pressure and the blackness inside of me. While I was surrounded by that strange splashing noiselessness, everything else was at peace.

Feeling into the young worker version of myself from that time, I sense my inability to recognize when I had hit *too much*. Crashing into a wall of exhaustion once more, I would wonder how it got there, how it snuck up on me so quickly again.

This was the beginning of learning my inner scale—the positive qualities of my experience balanced by those which were quietly injurious. One side of the scale held all my drive and fire, while the other side held my form, limp and lifeless. Life was offering me the opportunity to understand the difference between fluid passion and forced propulsion.

The myth of achieving some perfect life balance gets sucked into the storm of reality just when we think we have achieved it. There is really no such thing. But I do believe in some sensible in-between along this spectrum—at the other end of positive discipline, completion, manifestation, and full engagement lies some deep rest. How quick I was in the past to over-give of myself, to lean towards adrenal fatigue, thoughtless push, and an unconscious belief in some continuous struggle.

Women are allowed to have ambitions. But what really matters is the energy behind that ambition, its real fuel source. When ambition is whipped forward with a surface-level proving, a strong front of brute force, then we are relying on self-imposed aggression to get things done, which is the old patriarchal model.

This is to unconsciously believe that it always has to be hard. So many of us have taken this false belief and made it a fact in us: that we are not doing life right if it does not feel painful. But there does exist another way. When we touch into the true energy behind our ambition and let it be fed by trust in ourselves and the process—when it comes from genuine excitement and devotion—then we can move onwards with a more authentic motivation. We may realize that we don't need to push the river so damn hard all of the time.

This realization has helped me tune into my deep indoctrination of unconsciously thinking I can prove my worth through my doings. These strivings were quietly motivated by some persistent belief I could make my life "right" through less red ink on the page, a warm pat on the back, or a glowing comment from another human. In a world that can feel out of control, I was driven by the hope that I could "control" the ratcheting of my own doing. Somewhere along the way, I learned that being overwhelmed was normal, productivity was all-holy, and chronic busyness was the highest status symbol of all.

Entombed deep within the industrial age values of the current school system, as if in a factory, I learned that everyone must learn the same way. That my worth was based on memorization and jumping through hoops well. That there was no room left for genuine curiosity or to veer onto a course motivated by your own questioning. That learning happens through lecturing, studying, and taking exams—within a system where authority figures largely dictate how you spend your time, managing your "autonomy" for you.

I did my best to keep on pulling myself up by the bootstraps of my worker bee self within the system of the father principle. But when your life is filled up with math facts, papers on Christopher Columbus, and sports practice, there is no time for anything else.

I began to work solely for work's sake.

There is something spirit-sucking about the entire affair when we do not allow a young person to be seen for her own thoughts, delights, and soul, but directly aim to manipulate her life's path from the beginning. It is an aggression to lock up that child's wild nature, her dreams and her wonder, which are perhaps the ultimate expression of her true human potential.

What about wonder? Wonder gives us the eyes and hearts of two-year-olds engaging in a love affair with the natural world around them. When we wonder, we allow ourselves to be available, interested, open. We nurture and trust our own inquisitiveness. We whet our appetites for the quantum froth of mystery.

We feel possible to ourselves.

And it is in this self-possibility that we burst out of the constraints of our "factory settings" and let ourselves be more than "right" or "certain." Even more than "accomplished" or "successful," through possibility we sink into some kind of well of plenty that exists deep inside us. At which point, we may remember to put spirit first.

But in my swimming years, it was as if I was moving through the waters of my life with heavy anchors attached, always threatening to pull me into some starless and futile abyss. I knew nothing of the experience of healthy fullness. Like so many young women in their teenage years I knew of a stomach that was too full and then emptied, of the binging and purging cycle of a lack of integration. Of the hunger that is never satiated, never settled.

Unable to integrate the expectation of smooth perfection with what I was really feeling, I had not a core of sufficiency, but one of anxiety, depression, and inner pain. Through binging and purging I indulged in a repetitive, unfulfilling catharsis of the toxic black sludge of my emotions, like an endless spilling over.

I was wanting to be completely emptied out and scraped clean, yet this release, even the physical purging, never seemed enough. The dregs of this pain became like unexpressed and sticky hairballs, so hard to expectorate. Oh, how I admired the ease with which owls could cough up their pellets in little contained bundles.

By my early twenties, I had become anemic, physically and spiritually. My body was always being pushed, and I often felt dizzy or like I was walking at high altitude. I had a pit of loss, but no words to describe it, no skills to understand it. This inner anemia left me like a hollow reed. Parched, rattly, a shell of sorts with no nourished core.

As a young woman I was never taught, or I hadn't yet discovered, how to truly feed myself. I received cultural lessons in the importance of external appearances but did not know how to attend to my vital innards. I hadn't yet figured out what real nourishment was in ways that would fill my deep reserves, my heart and my spirit. I hadn't yet learned how to "rest" at the level that goes far beyond the culturally approved concept of lying around on the weekend.

Indoctrinated into an idea that more is always better, I believed more busyness meant more fullness—which meant more personal worth. I hadn't yet connected with a confidence that understands the purpose and place of both work and sprit, effort and rest, knowing when to act and when to be still.

There is no challenge more persistent and prevalent among women than the invisible, internal beliefs that lead them into life-long patterns of exhaustion, overwork, and overwhelm. Working themselves to the bone, all too often they fall into a dry and desolate wasteland of their own doing.

Patterns of unconscious proving are so ingrained that we may not recognize them at all anymore: proving through our overdoing, proving through our over-feeling, proving through our over-giving.

And on some level, we are straining to prove our fundamental worth and basic goodness. These provings are unreliable evidence to justify our place on this planet. They keep us striving just for the sake of it, distracted from aligning with our greater responsibility—the uncovering of our life's sacred instructions.

Embracing rest as a spiritual practice opens the possibility for soul-deep replenishment, restoration, and marrow-level renewal. Water as an element guides us into sinking into our own truths and learning to flow with the autonomous currents of our lives. For we will never know feminine confidence if we are chronically burned out and exhausted in our very centers. It is impossible for us to feel into saturated self-assurance when we are always depleted, running on the energetic equivalents of ashes and dust. Just as our physical bodies cry for energy, minerals and nutrients, our souls are crying for food— cardboard-like soul food is no longer enough.

The Left-over Scraps

There are so many ways that women are spiritually anemic, wandering the shallows of their lives. Busyness mimics the effect of a pack of cigarettes, a dull numbing of any real soul-appetite, covering up any cravings for something more, leaving us jangly and stimulated.

We think we can do it all: soothe the screaming baby, feed the whining dog, take the work call, do the core strengthening squats, and prep for dinner—while our hair stays coiffed and our lipstick fresh.

All too often we are putting ourselves on hold, allowing others' needs, problems, or desires to come before our own. I think of all of the examples of on-hold women I know, the mother who holds her bladder for a few hours past when she needs to go because she has a busy toddler who doesn't stop, or the nurse who skips her lunch because she has a demanding and lonely patient on floor three of the hospital, or the wife who doesn't even truly taste the beautiful dinner she prepared because she is no longer hungry, having spent the last two hours in the kitchen.

Deep down we know it injures us when we have to tamp down and quiet our own basic needs in order to serve another. The wrongness of it flickers in our bellies and nags at us. Of course, sometimes we are truly entrenched by circumstance. But other times we give generously and through willing agreement out of our longing to feel worthwhile through caring for another.

Even though we no longer live in an era when women are raised, groomed, and educated solely to perform the roles of wife and mother, the old roles women were constrained to play still are at work in the daughters and granddaughters of this time. It has been fed to us in the model of the ever-serving mother. Of the grandmother that is so busy taking care of others during the Thanksgiving holiday that she never sits down to eat herself.

This on-hold woman lives in all of us somewhere, a passed-down essence of a toxic giver. Unknowingly contagious, this archetypal energy is surprisingly harmful—a subtle disease passed from mother to daughter along with those bowls of potatoes.

How much is finally too much? A deep ambivalence gnaws away at us, a vast and confusing gray area takes hold as we love this giving but haven't quite figured out where its invisible but essential edges lay. Where are its boundaries? It is so easy to blow right through them, over-giving once more out of conditioning, habit, or strange comfort.

When I think of an over-giving woman, a mother octopus comes to mind. After laying her hatch of eggs she will cover her future brood with her body, not eating or leaving for a moment, ever ready to protect and defend. Her form will slowly pale, shrink, and deteriorate until by the time the eggs have hatched, death will have taken her. One octopus was documented caring for its young this way for a full fifty-three months. The biologist who studied this particular octopus described how "no mother could give more."[2]

But really how much should a mother give? Yes, protecting her future hatchlings is a mother octopus's biological imperative and we are not octopuses, but people. For us, it is an interesting metaphor, a splinter of a question to irritate our minds for a while.

As the philosopher and psychoanalyst Carl Jung, determined: "Nothing exerts a stronger psychic effect upon the human environment, especially upon children, than the life the parents have not lived."[3] On a buried unconscious level, our upbringings are the product of our parents' deep unfulfilled aspirations and sense of the world. When they felt like they had enough—enough resources, food, friends, love—they passed on this feeling. But when there was a sense of inner starvation, an embodied poverty—well, that got layered into us too.

Many of us are stuck in patterns of feeling for other people, whether it be our parents, our friends, or even the entire world. We may have learned long ago that we could feel much more in control of scary or stressful situations if we took over feeling for everyone around us. We may have unconsciously decided that if we took on their sadness, their angst, their fears, then we were doing something or helping in some way. Even as adults we may still believe in letting the heavy emotional detritus accumulate—gathering problems like tucked children under our skirts.

Important concerns, but not really ours.

And at some point, ten times heavier emotionally than we should be, we might get curious and start to wonder: *What would it feel like to let go of everyone else's feelings and just focus on my own?*

With or without realizing it, we are constantly being tasked to know where we focus our energy and to understand better what we cradle and make our own. With a flinty discernment, we can begin to perceive more accurately what holds true merit in our lives and what is really ours to give or feel. Finding clearer edges around these boundaries allows us to move lighter and more confidently through the world, no longer bogged down with all of the feelings and struggles of everyone around us. What have we been making our own?

It is not always so easy to catch when we are giving too much. But with the straightforward, discerning power of the Space Dancer, we might contemplate why we may tend to leave ourselves only the meager leftovers, the scraps of time, energy, and space. Taking out your journal, write on the following questions:

- *Are there any areas in your life where you over-give to prove your worth or your usefulness as a woman?*

- *What needs might you need to bring forward now, to be addressed at the front instead of the back of the line?*

Labyrinth of Distraction

Women have more freedoms and opportunities available to us than ever before, but instead of having these possibilities translate into more happiness and fulfillment, too often they become the "burden of more." This burden is the perpetual feeling of never having enough time, despite using your instant pot, smartphone scheduler, and multitasking upon multitasking. This is the all-consuming shroud of *constant doing* that covers up any chance for deeper connection with that wild, spirit-starved beast inside us.

The psychic heaviness of our schedules, responsibilities, obligations, accumulations, and expectations settles in our physical bodies right at the meeting point between our necks and upper backs. In traditional Chinese medicine there is an acupuncture point that rests right at this junction whose name translates as "one hundred labors." This is where many people, past and present, have carried their physical loads, such as water, firewood, or other supplies. This is where the yoke of a hardworking ox rests around its lower neck. And it is the place where we unconsciously stack up our many burdens of more.

It can be hard for us to perceive this load. The irony of our unrelenting busyness, with its speed and its distractions, is that it keeps us from tuning in to ourselves. As the pace just increases, we struggle to notice the weight we are carrying, oblivious of how the layers of our obligations accrue. But when we have brief moments of pause, a sickness, an injury, a vacation, or a lazy Sunday, we might have a slight glimpse into the mechanics of our self-created yokes. The chaffing of discomfort comes to our attention when we momentarily hold a clear gaze on our industry.

For women, this acupuncture point holds the energy of a special kind of labor; it is the holding place of so many doings. This is the hidden world of details, the things that so obediently lie still under the rug. When swept out into the open and gathered in the light, these doing things connect into a far-reaching web that forms the essential foundation for everything else in our lives.

This web is the gifts planned for the holidays, the knowing where the lost sock is hiding, the reminding about vitamins that need to be swallowed, the sending of birthday cards on time, and the hearing of the plants crying for water. It is "I Love You" notes stashed in lunches. It is the clean placemats laid out for steaming meals, the dishes scrubbed tidy, and the kisses given. It is so easy to take these small and ordinary things for granted, to assume these many hidden tasks will always be done. There is an accumulation effect to all these unacknowledged doings that women do, that adds value to daily life.

These doing things are beautiful and insignificant and sacred at the same time. I love them when I remember to see them as holy—when I don't have something boiling on the stove that demands my focus, or someone yelling for me, or some urgent place to be.

But because of the sheer number of things to do, pressure accumulates and it can be hard to see them as a spiritual practice.

Sometimes my response is to attempt to work faster and less mindfully. I allow these things to push me beyond my natural rhythm, adding to the speed that already swells in my life. This busyness distracts me from accessing the deeper layers of myself.

This is the dynamic that keeps us eternally scratching the surface.

Spiritual teacher Marianne Williamson writes: "Many of us have set up our lives so that we are constantly busy, living on a kind of adrenaline that poses as energy. This is an insidious trick of the negative mind: building a wall of frantic activity that mitigates the experience of a meaningful inner life."[4]

Take a breath here. You may feel like you need one.

In a way, all of this busyness is a tricky camouflage for the pain of negating your own needs—otherwise you would actually have to feel it: all the dissatisfaction, all the ways that your actions don't match your values, and the reality of your life flying by.

There are times when we are desperate to continue weaving our labyrinth of distractions. This unconscious coping mechanism saves us from truthfully facing a sucky job, an unsatisfying relationship, or even the presence of change itself. The hustle keeps us from feeling the more uncomfortable themes of life, like the truth of our existence, which is uncertainty, impermanence, and mortality.

Along with busyness and speed come a feeling of always being focused on the future. We unconsciously promote a sense that at some point down the road we'll be able to escape things *not being quite right*. We entertain all sorts of future thinking, such as:

When my children are grown, then . . .

When I start my new business, then . . .

When I leave this city, then . . .

Things will somehow be better.

The mind always moving a few steps in front of the body. But not being present grows a deep crevasse of anxiety within us.

The seeker, wearing herself ragged, feet bloodied with all of her searching, is always looking for more. She engages in the relentless pursuit to find validation and contentment outside of herself, somewhere down the line.

This begs the question: Who would we be without all that distraction, without all that speed?

Looking deeper allows us to see how our busyness addiction is just another version of the approval addiction, sneakily spiffed up. It acts as the sly accomplice of the ego, which is always trying to prove our worth through our efforts, success, and engagement. The worth and polish of our lives.

There is a kind of barrenness in our hearts when we are not tuning in. When the buffers we have placed on our perception are so thick that we can no longer hear the songs of our heartstrings vibrating. These are the times when I feel most lost, most anxious. When the busy walls of my life have no windows to look or escape through, and I feel captive in a prison of self-created frenzy.

We sidestep our personal power when we allow ourselves to be constantly lured away from our sense of spiritual connection. When the inner antlers of our spirit no longer point upward. When we are too much of this world.

So, what are the countermeasures?

We must be brave enough to look our fear of empty space square in the eyes. Without space to dream, feel into our intuition, and listen for our truths, we forget who we are. We must be continuously answering the call of this remembering.

We must take the cultural godliness out of busyness and stop worshipping it at its hurried source. Catching the ways we prop up a sense of importance and worth within ourselves, we must take responsibility for how we perpetuate this whir of doing.

We must let the living world remind us of the naturalness of our inner cycles. We are just not meant to act, engage, and project outwards all of the time. For between periods of blooming and growing come pauses of rest, opportunities for us to pull our energy down deep into our strong, expansive roots. Clarissa Pinkola Estés describes how the "psyches and the souls of women also have their own cycles and seasons of doing and solitude, running and staying, being involved and being removed, questing and resting, creating and incubating, being in the world and returning to the soul place."[5]

I love the reminder in her words: periods of reverent rest allow us to hear our soul's voice speaking. Laying ourselves down in waterways of restoration is not just for our weary bodies or overworked minds, but it provides us with essential opportunities to align with our soul's wisdom. And guided by feminine confidence, we dare allow ourselves this rest without guilt or shame. We respect and uphold the natural rhythms of our giving.

At times when I still get pulled into a whirlwind of busyness, sanity waits for me everywhere in nature. Looking around, I feel the lack of rush, the equanimity of the towering fir trees that line a nearby busy highway. I imagine them watching over the many passing cars and shaking their heads, baffled by the continuous human hustle.

Even in all of the things that seem rushed in nature—the push of a storm as it moves over the mountains or the rapids of a river as they run to the sea—there is some natural relaxation in their cadence. The elements all around me, air, earth, fire, and water, teach me to find their pulse of expansion and contraction, uncovering their organic flow within myself.

The element of air reminds me of aliveness as the crisp, green autumn winds blow through, merging and finding space between my atoms and the mesh of my fascia, ensuring that I too could lift off, I could become some other form of air.

The element of earth reminds me of rootedness as I walk through the forest, a messy room of leaves in wild disarray, beautiful and recalcitrant. The volatile oils of the trees enter my nose and fill my senses so that little shoots of wood begin to sprout and surge through me.

The element of fire reminds me of vitality as I watch a candle flicking its skirts, laughing and mischievous. Its life-giving glimmer is frisky, then smooth, undulating then steady. Its radiance of hope penetrates my heart, adding life force to all of the smaller fires within me, stoking the flares of my digestion, the pulsing of my blood vessels, and the spark of my neurons.

The element of water reminds me of freedom as afternoon ocean waves turn me into a devotee of sparkles, their light becoming liquid, my body becoming slippery, fluid, seal-like. This is the language of magic spoken in the bursts and tones of glitter. The waves know this prose, changing from pale green to turquoise and violet in the course of seconds, as they are shapeshifting from towering anticipation to crashing, frothy completion. And now my body remembers what it is to become water.

Connecting with the living world unites us with the force of nature that lives in and flows through us. We can follow this fresh, invigorating flux of vitality through everything and everyone, following a cloud until we are that cloud, feeling the sun until we are that light, lying in the grass until we have sunken and become one with the dirt.

Feeling into the sturdiness of feminine confidence, we cannot keep looking toward busyness to prove that our lives have meaning. All of this overdoing is a very fragile and untrustworthy method of connecting with our value. We must be diligent in catching and deciphering the ways in which we hide behind this rushing around to avoid feeling into our tender hearts.

With the insights of Wild Gaia and immersing ourselves within the living world, reflect on how to live a life that is fulfilling and not just full. With your journal in hand, let's explore further.

- *Study your own need to be busy. Observe how you reply when friends or relatives ask how you are doing; how often do you automatically respond with "Oh, I'm just really busy!"*

- *Through free writing, explore what restless fear might take hold if you stopped trying to prove yourself through your actions? How do you use busyness as a status symbol, as an unconscious argument in favor of your usefulness as a human?*

- *What does the living world have to teach you about using your energy more wisely? Reflect on the naturalness of your inner cycles and wonder about how you could tune in and honor them more.*

First Sink

Perhaps I have turned to water so much in my life because it is the opposite of fire. Because of all the times I have laid myself down in a dry creek bed of my own doing, some depleted and scorched version of myself, I have become accustomed to waiting for water. Every fall I watch trickles of water slowly fill summer crusted waterways, grateful to see the return of small water bugs and slick newts. And when exhaustion comes for me, I wait for my inner creek to fill, letting lifegiving water run around, over, and through me until I too am brought back to life again.

It is the fluid nature of water that makes it both a beginning and an end, a vessel of paradox. In traditional Chinese medicine, *zhi* is the spirit of the water element.

Every element contains an emotional/spiritual expression and zhi relates to our instinctual power or aligned will, or some might say, our confidence. When their zhi is imbalanced, people will continually push themselves to the point of total exhaustion, or on the flip side, they may have no motivation or initiative at all.

People sometimes use excessive amounts of caffeine, chemical stimulants, ambition, or desire to propel themselves forward. This can result in physical symptoms such as burnout, whole-body fatigue, insomnia, hormonal imbalances, chronic back pain, anxiety, or a total disintegration of the nervous system.

Because so many women are relying on their stress hormones to get them through their days, they don't have any clear sense of what their natural physical energy levels even are. They are really working from a "wired but tired" pattern. They are buzzing on the surface, burning through the push of cortisol, but underneath the busyness they are crispy fried.

As you might imagine, overwork is the number one reason for zhi imbalance, but other common causes include lack of sleep or poor sleep, excessive physical activity, chronic pain or disease, chronic fear, residuals of childhood trauma, and multiple births and/or an excessive loss of blood during periods. So many people on our planet are in a state of zhi disturbance.

Water contains a dual nature, holding the polarities of both yin and yang. Because of its fluid shapeshifting, it endlessly gives birth to its own opposite. It is what seems impossible, the yin fire that sparks the mysterious potency of matter. It knows how to receive and hold (yin), then intensely move and give (yang). It is the nourishing quality of the uterus to cradle a growing baby (yin), but it is also the tremendous pushing force with which it thrusts that baby out (yang). It is the burst of the shooting star (yang) across the jet black of the new moon sky (yin)—powerful movement that erupts from complete stillness.

The healing process of bringing the zhi into balance requires returning to the mystery of water, like a stone that gets dropped into the still, purple waters of a pond deep in an unknown forest. For it is in nature that we can slow long enough to begin to sink like a stone. We can finally let our overworked arms learn to be open. Laying slack, just hanging there. Letting our bodies sink like rocks to the very bottom of that dark purple lake, tiny bubbles arising as we fall.

In meditation, I watch myself . . .

drop,

   drop,

      drop,

         until I land softly on the sandy floor.

The settled stone of me just sits on all my noise, opinions, and distractions, allowing my true senses to sharpen into the pointed tip of discernment and presence. While everything else is getting heavy, my mind is getting lighter, sharper, more crystalline. I feel all of life around me in brighter colors, more animated, and electric.

I am here, just here. Letting my agenda slide away, too slippery to catch.

In its place rests a trust in myself just as I am.

There is sweetness in being left with so little.

As acupuncturist Lori Eve Dechar describes: "Here the light of consciousness is buried in darkness and the spirits bathe in the underworld waters of the unconscious. Here the lights of the spirits wait, like the nutrients and minerals waiting in the soil, until the goddess releases them back into the life cycle to nourish new psychic structures."[6] In her words, I feel the potency of what is waiting for us in the dark stillness, the sustenance that wants to be released.

There is an art to engaging in spiritual rest, knowing when to withdraw in order to enter life more fully. Learning to pull our energy in is like the ocean pulling in her waves, gathering herself with a brief pause before releasing her charge once more. The ocean knows how to move inwards before forging outwards. She is not a relentless, thrusting force of propulsion, a crash, crash, crash. I imagine how destructive and insatiable she would be, only moving forward this way. But so often this is how we are interacting with our world, a damaging, distracted tsunami that consumes and engages with no rest, no peace, no listening.

Among the Australian Aboriginal peoples, there is a state of being known as *dadirri,* a term that translates as "deep listening."[7] Miriam Rose Ungunmerr-Baumann, an Australian Aboriginal elder, describes dadirri as a special quality that allows each of us to make contact with a rich spring that lies within us. When we connect from this state of quiet awareness, it offers us a chance to renew ourselves psychically and spiritually.

Amazingly, it is thought that some form of dadirri has been practiced by humans for over 40,000 years—since the Paleolithic era. The truth is that many cultures throughout history have engaged in some kind of similar practice. As we match the energy of the living world around us, we slow to notice all of the sensations, sounds, and smells, taking the time to listen to all creation breathe. Pulse. Vibrate.

Sitting by the soft purl of a river, you can allow your own creativity and imagination to float and swell.

You can know ease.

Lying in the golden husks of late-summer grasses, you can fill yourself up with simple observations, taking in the mastery and agility of a cobalt swallow feeding in midair.

You can know awe.

Resting in the primordial intelligence and dynamic flux of the universe, you can remember that you are spirit-made-flesh, stunning and also completely insignificant.

You can know astonishment.

The word *astonish* comes from the Latin *extonare,* which means "to thunder," to shake with sudden wonder.[8] To be rattled with disbelief. To feel struck and blown over by the enormity of it all—the cosmos, the magic, the mystery—while resting in the soft womb of the holy unknown.

We can no longer use our will, our ego, our push, our drive to resolve the problem of busyness. We cannot pass our troubles off to someone else, hoping that some guru, some healthcare practitioner, some doctor or acupuncturist will fix it for us. If this is an issue you struggle with, at long last you are asked to hold your hands up in a peace offering, to fully acquiesce to your need for rest and renewal. Beginning the process of restoration begins with sensing an uncontainable yearning for something different for yourself.

Sometimes we have to learn this the hard way. In my case, this has meant periods of exhaustion and forced rest. Others may feel it as being fed-up with always stuffing their soul-longings down, weary of feeling tuned out from their primal longings, sick and tired of their constant speed.

The truth is that when we are moving continuously, we don't find out what we are moving from. When we sit still, in meditation, contemplation, or prayer, we can honestly experience where we are.

For it is in this stillness that our truths get whispered. Here we grope in the dark, studying our edges and borderlands, learning how to feel into ourselves with grace and compassion. Allowing ourselves this time in the unknown without immediately trying to change it, fix it, or cover it is to take a great pause, to work with the medicine that comes from a watchful suspension of all doing.

We are being told to sit on the bottom of the forest pond now, to rest in its void and fully let the gravity of our sinking penetrate us. This is an opportunity to honestly view how we may have been sacrificing ourselves, inauthentically using the power of our will. This moment is an opportunity to engage in an alchemical process, to use our experience of exhaustion or overload to initiate real change in our lives and, allowing for the blooming of a healthy confidence that is based first in rest, then in action.

Our Inner Healer asks us not to use distractions and speed to stand in the way of hearing our deeper wisdom; we must pause so that we can hear when we are being asked to make dramatic and lasting revisions to our way of life. Using your journal again, here are some contemplations.

- *Imagining myself sunken to the bottom of a still purple pond is one of my favorite meditations when I am feeling tired to the bone. Experiment with feeling into the healing power of the water element when you are needing a great pause. Pull in all of the sensorial details: the color of the water, the feel of it on your skin, the peace of the noiselessness, the heaviness of your body.*

- *Our souls know nothing of the language of busyness, distraction, and speed. What does your soul want to tell you about resisting the seductive pull of constant doing?*

- *How does sitting still with the sufficiency of yourself relate to feeling a different, more grounded kind of confidence? With solid energy powering your core, how does this make your confidence feel more unshakeable?*

Trust in Your River

As you can tell by all the water that has already flowed through these pages, my whole life I have been obsessed with being an underwater creature. At ten, I would squeeze both of my feet into the opening of one swimming flipper, squirmy in their union. My child's mind could initiate the transformation of flesh into scales, mermaid skin spreading over my boney leg gap. I loved plunging and swaying with the currents of the water, and the mixing of temperatures, never being entirely sure if I was up or down. Then I would find the water's edge, my lone flipper smacking the surface for effect. I thought I was mystical.

Gradually this flurry of effort would wane, as my legs would grow heavy and I would sink toward the bottom of the pool, listless.

"Dead" but very awake.

And then I would carefully inspect every otherworldly treasure I could find: a wad of gum, a soggy Band-Aid, a forgotten hair-tie. A time machine seemed to grab the seconds and hold them back, hypnotizing them into something drunk and docile. Infused with a muffled peace, the dreamscape of this water world offered me a pause, an antidote to the aggressive marching of time gone by. My coral lungs could expand and vibrate, finding a truce from my everyday existence.

Again and again, I returned to the secret underwater world in pools and lakes and oceans. Really in any kind of water I could find. I found an ease there, even in the crushing moments of a wave pinning me down, skin rubbed raw in the sand at the seashore. Peace was there, even in the inky black of the lake, obese and secretive, threatening to keep me in its weedy tendrils. It was there in the clear waters, too, sparkly and compelling, a collection of light flecks and bubbles.

So many years later, I still visit the water world, although less often and with no flippers. I still love to rest my belly on the bottom of a pool and listen. But with time I have learned to be curious about opposites and I have also taken to playing above the surface. I have taken to floating, resting with my face toward the sky, my ears still in the water, intaking my own loud breathing. The echo chamber of my blood beating the drum of my pulse in my ears. Alien and intimate. This is the breath and blood of a child, young woman, and adult mother. I find all of myself here, in the hover of belonging.

Occasionally as I float on this windowpane of water, the glassy surface will be unexpectedly broken by summer raindrops dancing like little fingertips musically touching the surface of my flesh and the skin of the water. Rain will pitter on my face, creating a reflex of blinks. The drops sing of change and the unrestrained movement of nature. The simplicity of the moment has the effect of expansion, ripples upon ripples, into more ripples.

The water in my own cells want in on this evolution, these circles dancing with each other, water everywhere, inward, outward, above

and below. I feel all of the past and the future in this brief coalescing—
the barriers of separation dissolving away. Yes, I am still mystical.

With my adult imagination, I see the barrier of this pool break open,
a levee gone mad. Out of it flows the great river of my life, and I am
awash in its currents, picking up speed, just barely remembering how
to swim.

This river knows me and my tricks.

It knows how I long to control, my white knuckles clenched in
distrust and false control. These waters submerge me and toss me over
while asking: Who are you, really? Who are you when you live for
yourself, with the voice of your soul leading the way? When your soul's
life is your truest responsibility?

The great river of my life encourages me to know my own authority
as a woman. Beyond the invisible tethers of family, culture, and society.
It moves me to find depth in my questions and answers. Often the
water is docile enough for me to take in a quick breath before
submerging again. I hope there will be air to breathe soon.

I have forgotten how to rest in the tides with all of my adult
pushing, striving, and doing. So much worry and weight. This river is
merciful but relentless. It encourages me to lose "myself" in all kinds
of experiences. To allow for the creative ebb and flow of everything.

My early water training serves me well here. I call upon that girl
within, the mermaid creature who loves to swim. She has never died
in self-doubt. She teaches me about confidence, sovereignty, and
mystery. The gentleness of being cradled. She feels the rapture of being
a nature spirit, reminding me to turn over onto my back.

No, you won't drown.

She asks me to remember that there is a sky up there with paths of
stars, the light-filled pinpricks of heaven's lace, that guide the way. She
holds my hand as we glide along and then she whispers in my ear: *trust
in this river.*

As women we must learn to trust in the river of our lives. To trust its movement, its curves and currents, its autonomous flow.

This trust asks us how much we have been relying on survival mode? It asks what percentage of each day our cells get the message to be tense soldiers instead of dancers of biological beauty.

Trust is not a thoughtless acquiesce or a passive faith that things will easily flow your way. It is an empowered surrender as an active participant, fueled by courage and action versus apathetically wishing things were different.

Trusting, softening, unraveling can be downright terrifying. Despite wanting to trust and desperately yearning to lay our bodies down in the posture of prostration, head touching the ground, often our cells, muscles, and mental doings turn reflexively toward defensiveness. Over time, this feeling of being tense and restricted wants to move from the mental-emotional realm and trickle into our physical form. Tension creeps into tissues of our bodies, the connective sheets and fascial layers turned into compressed, shrink-wrapped guarding.

Trust is persuasive, gently coaxing your body to rest, every time your spine gets rigid and your head pops up from sleep. Trust reminds you to unclench your fingers, let your belly grow supple, let your traps unravel, and let your jaw hang low. It convinces all your receptacles of tension to unfurl and flow.

The birthing process teaches this trust for a mother always dilates more than she contracts. She expands her physical body further than she ever thought possible to allow for her child's essence (and huge head) to move from the fluid, trustworthy, watery world of the womb to the solid, earthly external world. Just like a mother in the becoming, we must birth new possibilities within ourselves.

Call it expansion, call it personal evolution, call it faith—trust is the greatest softener I know. I am brought back time and time again to this trust, a trust in the river of my life.

I have always been drawn to the Earth with its biting white peaks, clumsy piles of boulders, crimson canyonlands, and knife-sliced basalt cliffs. I have searched my entire life for ground. For stability, safety, security. For feet pressed in sacred dust and body laid in wet, enveloping grass.

I guess you could say I was unconsciously searching for the comfort of something impervious to pain. And who doesn't want that really? But over time I began to perceive what all of this predictability was doing to me. That pretend certainty was not really my friend all along.

I was mistaking comfort as true joy.

I realized I am not here to be safe. Perhaps instead I am, as we all are, here to risk it all.

Searching for comfort was its own trap. Its own lumbering, heavy weight. A block to truth.

I still love to feel myself as an Earth-being, but I have become more open to water and the way it wants to shape and carve and move through my earth.

I have become available—no, dedicated—to my beautiful erosion.

There is this water of enhanced flexibility and fluidity that wants to work on me now. Something always moving in me.

It is the natural strength in this river of inner trust that is the true core of feminine confidence. The waters of trust flow within you, always longing to return to their source. Back to the throat, back to the heart, back to the womb, back to the blood, back to the marrow, back to the DNA strands, back to your sorrow, back to your fear, back to your enlightenment, back, back, further, to remembering where you've come from. These hidden waters are the keepers of your memories.

Let the long, flowing dawdlings of trust work through you now, washing from the crown of your head down through every microscopic opening all the way to your toes. This rebellious inner relaxation will tell you that it has long since given up its search party for security and certainty. They are dead to her now.

Just in case you have forgotten, laying in the hand of trust reminds you that you are already doing "it." Already doing everything you are meant to do. And that there exists an inherent completeness to you, right now, in this moment.

Your life, cunning teacher that it is, will continue to lead you.

Using the intuitive strength of your Inner Healer, imagine how life's external factors, the fears and challenges you encounter offer you opportunities to retrain yourself in trust instead of further tightening down. Use your journal right now to explore trusting in the river of your life.

- *Reflect and connect with this river. Free write or draw what it looks like, texturally exploring its flow, its curves, its rapids. Experiment using images of water to feel into your wild autonomy and free expression. How would it feel to lay down in this river?*

- *One of the most profound acts of trust I have ever witnessed was in Tibet, watching Buddhist pilgrims complete hundreds and hundreds of prostrations and prayers, so many that they would wear calluses on their foreheads from where their heads touched the ground. Over and over again they moved with devotion, letting their bodies and minds be completely emptied out of everything except trust. As a humble act of trust, experiment with a daily practice of touching your head to the floor or the ground, as a simple commitment to trust in your life.*

- *Contemplate (or write about) how a daily engagement and cultivation of trust in yourself leads to and connects you with an essential, unshakable kind of confidence.*

New Every Day

The incense is going. The candle is lit.

It is here in the early morning that I can pause in the familiar hammock of darkness. I follow the simplicity of my in-breath—*life*—and out-breath—*death*.

I am nothing more than flesh hanging on bones, the draped cloth of my skin less and less precise with every passing day. My anonymous skeleton floats in space, the living paradox of rarity and irrelevance, just like so many other beings on this planet.

Then all form disappears, and I can only perceive myself as a spiraling ball of light and energy, my resonance melding with that of the Earth and the great, sweeping mystery.

My attention shifts again, awakened by the raucous party of birds outside, shouting their joys through the window.

I home in on their sharp, repetitive notes, which are then interrupted by . . .

"Mommy, can I look at your phone to see the weather?"

My son's eyes are big and sincere, and I feel his sweetness in my cells. A simple request. Yet a space violation, initiating a rapid flood of resentment. In my mind, I imagine what it would be like to respond like an angry monster, its teeth gnashing. "This is my time," I would growl.

But that wouldn't be a very helpful, so I just take another breath before launching any arrows. This is the holding of space for the deep love and sufficiency of mothering mixed with the ambivalence, the fatigue of constant need meeting.

Then the other child comes in.

"Mommy, can you stretch out my pants? They don't feel good."

And so, the morning begins.

This is my daily practice. And honestly, I would lock the door, but they would just bang on it if I did. Believe me, I have tried. Rules and guidelines become fluid at the beginning of school-day mornings. So, I just wake up earlier and ease into this gray area, this messy, quasi-alone, ending-too-soon time.

I give you these humorous but true details to make a point: Your daily practice of spiritual rest and connection does not have to be perfect. Or crazy long. Or even uninterrupted for that matter.

But it does have to happen in a regular way. There is no way around the necessity of positive discipline and consistency. We must have an antidote to the relentless doings of our days, an opportunity to be still, go inward, and befriend ourselves.

Our feminine confidence is repetitively strengthened in simple acts of coming home to ourselves.

When I unabashedly choose myself, despite the activity of a hectic household, it is an act of true self-care and self-loyalty. Not self-care in all of its consumeristic, surface-scratching versions, but a self-care that directly links me to my soul. It is an expression that I value taking care of myself in this way more than any other activity in my life; I recognize its worth in spiritual gold.

We have a need for sacred connection and to know the forgiveness of being born new every day. The just-birthed sun shares its rising rays—wondrous shafts of freshness and revival—that then shine through the suns of our hearts. These red-drum wonders will hold their loyal rhythm for thousands of new beats in our chests over the course of this beautiful unfolding day.

With every morning, a bath of self-love is available to wash away the residue of all our previous shortcomings, unkept promises, and disappointments. This is an actual rebirth, not just a belief in it. This baptism of sweet gratitude for life lets you start all over again.

Every single day of our lives we make choices—some more conscious than others. Some are active decisions about how we shall speak, act, and use our time and energy. Often, however, we are living from a place of thoughtlessness or ingrained reactivity. Out of the thousands of fleeting thoughts that we experience every day, the vast majority of them are the same that we had the previous day. They are conditioned responses based on our limiting belief systems or reflexive behaviors.[9] Every day when we wake anew, our practice gives us the opportunity to live more consciously.

A helpful metaphor was once described to me about the purpose and effects of daily spiritual practice. Now imagine in your mind's eye that there is a huge mountain in your view that represents your sacred responsibilities. An overgrown forest lies between you and this mountain. You try to squeeze past all the overgrown brambles, the tree limbs and the endless vegetation, but it is very slow going.

The journey feels restrictive and frustrating and you often lose momentum or want to throw up your hands and turn around. But when you have a practice, it's like you have been suddenly gifted with a very sharp machete. The machete helps you to cut through old patterns and stories, to be the gentle, silent observer of your thoughts, to know yourself better every day. A practice helps you clear and track old patterns and behaviors, like a continuous house cleaning, preventing thick layers of emotional build-up from occurring.

What is a practice exactly? Oh, it can be so many things, meditation, prayer, contemplative activities, writing, the list really goes on and on. A practice is a space of creative connection designed by you. It is a time when you are inhabiting yourself fully.

Perhaps if you are a beginner a little more structure can be beneficial. But after over two decades of engaging with a regular meditation practice, I am less and less convinced that we have to pigeon-hole our practices into looking a certain way. Inner stillness, yes. Breath, yes. Open heart, yes. Gratitude, yes.

And an opportunity to engage with our internal compassionate observer. Your compassionate observer is that merciful witness inside that just watches. With judgeless observation, mind chatter becomes less gripping and all-powerful than it once was. The compassionate observer knows that on some days she will feel great, exalted with passion and clarity, while on other days she will feel puffy, hung over, ten pounds heavier, and ten years older—and she knows that this, too, shall pass.

Inviting ourselves into the model of the living world, we can remember that we are constantly changing, dying, growing, reborn. Even in the places we are shut down, there is always something living in us. Even after a devastating forest fire there are seeds waiting in the charred but fertile soil. If we look toward our vastly competent planet, we see that she has so many moods, so many outfits, so many ways that she is constantly changing and reinventing herself. Our task is learning not to reject any of it. To expand our sense of availability further and further out to make room for it all.

More than anything, compassionate observation is a practice in just that: self-compassion. It is a gentle witnessing, letting go of our inner evaluating in order to listen and observe without constantly flexing our mental claws. What a relief to release the hooks of our oh-so-very-important opinions, perceptions, and thoughts.

Imagine sitting on a lawn chair in the depths of summer, watching the movement of the clouds, morphing from a detailed fish into a wild dragon into a tangled mess of white threads floating away. Our thoughts also feel so permanent, so real and firm. But if we stick with them, we realize that just like the clouds, their power fades as their clear outlines begin to meld and dance in some ephemeral, fluid nature.

Sometimes we have come to a spiritual practice seeking relaxation or to zone out or find a way out of some grinding pain. But what we may realize is missing in the marketing of meditation as a stress management tool is genuine soul connection time.

In learning to listen to the language of our souls, we train in relating to ourselves and our world in a different way. Remembering that we are more than our physical bodies, we are reminded that the material constraints of our everyday lives are not so solid. Agreeing to a more multidimensional viewpoint, we are able to remember the impermanence of our short lives and the vast cycles at work within us and around us.

That zillions of star particles blissfully collided to make you as their living joy. You are the holy debris of this unbelievable confluence, made of the same miracles as elephants, earth worms, electric eels, and Everest. Ten sextillion atoms in the oxygen you breathe will have been shared by every person and creature alive and dead. Yes, you have been breathing the shared atoms of Joan of Arc and Cleopatra and Rosa Parks all along.

A regular practice of soul listening brings you back to the confidence of the instinctual woman. She sees the movement of your life intertwined in the movement of all living things. Along with the compassionate observer, she has a constant ear out for the messages of her inner truth. She is able to sit within the eye of her storm and just watch everything whirling about her. Being still, over and over again, despite all of the difficulties of life teaches us to stay, to witness, to trust.

As many times as you need to, as many mornings you are blessed to wake, you can always begin again.

Your Inner Healer knows what you need to stay spiritually grounded and connected. Here are a few more questions to consider in your journal.

- *If you do not have a regular practice of stillness, meditation, or reflection, take a moment to wonder about the barriers that stand in the way of you establishing a regular, committed practice? If you do have a practice, reflect on how this is the highest form of self-care.*

- *Experiment with gently connecting with the viewpoint of the compassionate observer. Becoming your own kind witness is a fierce and loyal action that returns you to feminine confidence.*

May you know your essential worth and goodness beyond the ways in which you may overdo, over-feel, or over-give—you have nothing left to prove.

May you come to see the way an addiction to busyness attempts to keep you detached from your personal power and deaf to your soul's voice.

May you gather healthy amounts of time, energy, creativity, and rest for yourself, knowing the confidence and vitality that come from prioritizing soulful self-care.

May you return to the freeing, healing, baptizing nature of water whenever you need to renew and revitalize your essence.

May you lay down in your own sacred waterway to relax in its currents and believe wholeheartedly in its autonomous nature. May you trust completely in the flow of your life.

ENDINGS AND BEGINNINGS

Every single day, about 1,800 thunderstorms dramatically reverberate across the planet. Sound waves from these storms bounce off the Earth's atmosphere and then echo in ripples around us. When we get cornered by one of these tempests it can feel like entering another world, a queendom of electrical impulses, undulating vibrations, savage energy, pressure, and power.

We may think that these storms are very much outside of us. But feeling into our own bodies, we can recognize many of the same elements: vibration, sound, electricity, and impulse. Our trillions of human cells are literally designed to conduct currents of power. In fact, it is the electricity that channels through our nervous systems that makes it possible for us to move, think, and feel. Our own devoted hearts, beating an average of 115,000 times per day, also speak the language of electricity and booms.

There is a storm in you too. Draw in the taste of its earthy freshness. Let its trembling force invigorate you. This is not a passing, temperamental squall but your storm of truth. Tumbling piles of flinty blue want to wash over you with unyielding liberation. Clouds of self-honesty act to transform your unexamined confidence into something more empowered, settled, and familiar. Lightning may bring you brief shocks of illumination or transient insight, but it is the rumbling power of thunder that reverberates and lingers in your marrow. The impulses of its sound vibrations resonate through your chest, shiver down your spine, put your little arm hairs on end, leaving you altered. Just let this storm of feminine confidence keep working within you.

At times, we may still be tempted to orient ourselves in the world through old styles of expressing confidence. This training runs deep in our default ways of being. Each time this happens, we must catch how we attempt to reinforce and perpetuate an unhealthy and self-limiting model within the spheres of our thinking and being. This obsolete model was based on the insecure wielding of power and weight—we don't need that anymore. Something you have to push out in front of you—we don't need that either.

The truth is that you do not have to feel confident every moment of your day to be in touch with your feminine confidence. You do not have to have banished every last bit of uncertainty or confusion from your life to still believe in your wholeness. Let us pull these vulnerabilities, these imperfections, these tangled strands of ourselves even closer. Instead of thinking we can exile, hide, or smother these experiences, let us hold them tighter. Let the mess of ourselves be part of our home turf. Instead of always looking for something purer to work with, let us stick with where we are.

Fighting off our urge for continuous improvement, ease, and comfort, let us bring all of the things that make us feel so far from confidence and let them be our wisdom teachers. When we learn to make space for all of our experience, we train ourselves in allowing in our honest feelings without letting them permanently rule us in stuckness. Instead, we can let them remind us of softening, everyday softer still with each act of self-compassion and trust.

For it is okay to have doubt or fear or dread. Lean into those feelings, letting your forehead touch doubt's forehead, letting your nose touch fear's nose, letting your lips touch dread's lips. And then walk on. You must walk on.

One foot trustingly placed in front of the other.

What I have learned about feminine confidence is that as you breathe it, live it, believe it, and continue to let it quicken within you organically, it begins to take on a life of its own. You do not need to know what it already all looks like. Walk forward anyway.

Talking, talking, talking will get us nowhere—now it is time to act. You choose with your actions. You choose with what words you feed yourself, you choose how you react, you choose how you birth yourself anew every day. Use the power of your conscious choice to understand very clearly what you return to within yourself. Feminine confidence is a series of repeated choices towards a resilient, persistent self-loyalty.

I feel a quickening in this age we live in, a sense of urgency, an acceleration of shift. The transformation of these times is not some magical, shiny reimaging of ourselves, but more of a decomposition. Things are ending and holding on tighter will do no good. Even when we don't know what is coming next, don't hold on. Just say yes—yes to the ending, yes to the falling away, yes to the decay of the old, worn-out energy that we have been immersed in. We must let go of what we no longer need so that we can share ourselves more fully with the world.

Deeply tired and bored of returning to the same stale and damaging patterns that keep us encaged and muzzled, now is not a time for smallness. You have a right to be here, to take up space, to have a voice. No more wallowing in insignificance, no more hiding out, no more invisibility. Treat your autonomy as its own religious practice. Let your own force of nature flow through you more freely now. Let it make you feel all stirred up. Agitated. Questioning. Wanting more.

Let your storm of truth keep moving you. Shifting its weight and restless with pressure, this thunder vows to keep you provoked. It draws you to it with a primal magnetism, the iron flecks in your heart drawing you towards its brewing moodiness. Feel the sky, thick with piles of black, shadowy beings rolling over each other, fractals of light piercing the spaces between their bodies. Life sustaining water is coming. A balance of energy and electricity is approaching. Fire sparked in the dark threatens with an unmistakable roar. Storm wisdom brings things to a head, clears the air, relaxes the energy, and readies us for something new.

We long to touch this wild, in ourselves, outside of ourselves. We yearn to feel a part of something so free. The transformational peal of thunder wants to jerk us out of complacency again and again, shocking us with aliveness, stirring us to inhabit our days with complete self-possession.

When we throw down the thunder of our confidence, this is not a display of personal power or forced proving. It is not yet another way to grasp power or to seek it outside of ourselves. Wielding our thunder well means that we are listening to and encouraged by what is untamed, hungry, and roaming in us.

We can no longer be afraid of what is raw and real—we can't afford to suppress this part of ourselves anymore. For in this era of the collective wake-up call, there is no more time to hold ourselves back—pulsing in the center of our storm is feminine confidence, our fiercest, softest, most natural state of being.

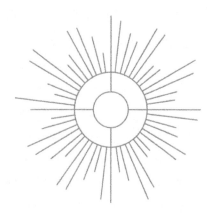

DEEP BOWS

"Your little will can't do anything. It takes Great Determination. Great Determination doesn't mean just making an effort. It means the whole universe is behind you and with you—the birds, trees, sky, moon, and ten directions."[1]
—KATAGIRI ROSHI

First bows: to the land.

I have to admit that in the beginning I thought I was walking through her. It was only in the repetition of the returning that the truth became clear—it was really the forest wandering through me, a firm nurse applying her salve to my heart.

The many fractals and tones of green from this land have healed something tender and quiet within me. Deep gratitude to Swordfern and Towhee, and all of the wise beings that have taught and continue to teach me through their very presence, all the way from the elder Sequoia to the vast cosmos of organisms living in the dark beneath my feet. This land has tucked me within her folds and reminded me that I am one of her own.

Thanks to my ancestors who continually beat their drums for me, those that lived well and died well, and who left wide footsteps for me to walk within. Thanks to the primordial powers, the sacred directions, the elemental powers, the seasons, and rhythms that put me back in place and remind me that I am not alone in the task of living.

Bows to my parents, Thomas Ward, Jr., and Nancy Angus-Edge, who both taught me to love the natural world in their own beautiful, unique ways.

Bows to all of those who provided a continual stream of love and encouragement along the way, Cherri Gallison, Christopher Ward, Campbell Van Plantinga, and my sisters of the Virgo Circle, Leah Vandenberg and Kristin Kuhn.

Bows to all of my patients over the years who have inspired these writings and who willingly trusted me with their most tender joys, pains, and vulnerabilities. It has been my gift to witness the bravery of your healing journeys.

Bows to Jara Kern, whose kindness and organizational genius helped so much in the early days of writing. Gigantic thanks to Jen Violi for the creativity boosts and developmental coaching. And humongous, whole-body prostrations to Stephanie Gunning, editor extraordinaire and friend, who helped me in so many ways during the writing of this book that I could not even list them all here. Thank you for graciously leading me through the dark unknown of this first book.

Bows to all of the causes and conditions that led to me to having the time and space to write for the love of it—I am a blessed woman. Thanks to my sun, Ansel, and my moon, Selene, for teaching me about the true nature of love. You create the warp and weft of my solar system. And love-drenched bows to my earth, Igor, for your endless support and encouragement, and for unquestioningly giving me the space I need to stretch my own wild spirit.

One of the great pleasures I enjoyed while writing this book was reading diverse source material. If you want to go further, I recommend the following books wholeheartedly.

Voices of the Body

Being Bodies: Buddhist Women on the Paradox of Embodiment, edited by Lenore Friedman and Susan Moon

Wild Feminine: Finding Power, Spirit and Joy in the Female Body, Tami Lynn Kent

The Beauty Myth: How Images of Beauty Are Used Against Women, Naomi Wolf

The Body Is Not an Apology: The Power of Radical Self-Love, Sonya Renee Taylor

Buddhist-Based Wisdom

Dakini Power: Twelve Extraordinary Women Shaping the Transmission of Tibetan Buddhism in the West, Michaela Haas

Wisdom Rising: Journey into the Mandala of the Empowered Feminine, Lama Tsultrim Allione

Standing at the Edge: Finding Freedom Where Fear and Courage Meet, Joan Halifax

The Way of Tenderness: Awakening Through Race, Sexuality, and Gender, Zenju Earthlyn Manuel

Opening the Lotus: A Woman's Guide to Buddhism, Sandy Boucher
When Things Fall Apart: Heart Advice for Difficult Times, Pema Chödrön

Spirit of a Woman

Women Who Run with the Wolves: Myths and Stories of the Wild Woman Archetype, Clarissa Pinkola Estes

Your Story Is Your Power: Free Your Feminine Voice, Susie Herrick and Elle Luna

If Women Rose Rooted: The Journey to Authenticity and Belonging, Sharon Blackie

Feminine Genius: The Provocative Path to Waking Up and Turning on the Wisdom of Being a Woman, LiYana Silver

Awaken Your Inner Fire: Ignite Your Passion, Find Your Purpose, and Create the Life That You Love, HeatherAsh Amara

Wild Embers: Poems of Rebellion, Fire, and Beauty, Nikita Gill

Rise Sister Rise: A Guide to Unleashing the Wise, Wild Woman Within, Rebecca Campbell

Burning Woman, Lucy Pearce

Wild Mercy: Living the Fierce and Tender Wisdom of the Women Mystics, Mirabai Starr

Belonging: Remembering Ourselves Home, Toko-pa Turner

Strong Is the New Pretty: A Celebration of Girls Being Themselves, Kate T. Parker

Good Night Stories for Rebel Girls, Elena Favilli

The Living World

Woman and Nature: The Roaring Inside Her, Susan Griffin

Reclaiming the Wild Soul: How Earth's Landscapes Restore Us to Wholeness, Mary Reynolds Thompson

Braiding Sweetgrass: Indigenous Wisdom, Scientific Knowledge, and the Teachings of Plants, Robin Wall Kimmerer

Conversations with Trees: An Intimate Ecology, Stephanie Kaza

Intimate Nature: The Bond Between Women and Animals, edited by Linda Hogan, Deena Metzger, and Brenda Peterson

Sisters of the Earth: Women's Prose and Poetry about Nature, Lorraine Anderson

Dwellings: A Spiritual History of the Living World, Linda Hogan

Underland: A Deep Time Journey, Robert MacFarlane

Voice of the Earth: An Exploration of Ecopsychology, Theodore Roszak

Uprising for the Earth: Reconnecting Culture with Nature, Osprey Orielle Lake

Soulcraft: Crossing into the Mysteries of Nature and Psyche, Bill Plotkin

Spiritual Ecology: The Cry of the Earth, edited by Llewellyn Vaughan-Lee

Rewilding: Meditations, Practices, and Skills for Awakening in Nature, Micah Mortali

Becoming Animal: An Earthly Cosmology, David Abram

The Wakeful World: Mind, Animism, and the Self in Nature, Emma Restall Orr

World as Lover, World as Self: Courage for Global Justice and Planetary Renewal, Joanna Macy

NOTES

Chapter 1: Feminine Confidence

[1] Clarissa Pinkola Estés, *Women Who Run with the Wolves: Myths and Stories of the Wild Woman Archetype* (New York: Ballantine Books, 1992), pp. 25–6.

[2] "Confidence (n.)," Etymonline.com (accessed June 21, 2019).

[3] Philip Ball. *Patterns in Nature: Why the Natural World Looks the Way It Does* (Chicago, IL.: University of Chicago Press, 2016), pp. 80–3.

Chapter 2: Storm of Inquiry

[1] Terry Tempest Williams, *When Women Were Birds: Fifty-four Variations on Voice* (New York: Picador, 2013), p. 225.

[2] "Confident," Powerthesaurus.org (accessed September 17, 2019).

[3] Anand Giridharadas, as cited in Elle Luna and Susie Herrick. *Your Story Is Your Power: Free Your Feminine Voice* (New York: Workman Publishing, 2018), p. 112.

[4] Susan Cain. *Quiet: The Power of Introverts in a World That Can't Stop Talking* (New York: Crown Publishers, 2012), p. 4.

[5] Scilla Elworthy. *Power and Sex: Developing Inner Strength to Deal with the World* (Dorset, U.K.: Element Books, 1997).

Chapter 3: Sovereign Natives

[1] Rebecca Campbell. *Rise Sister Rise: A Guide to Unleashing the Wise, Wild Woman Within* (Carlsbad, CA: Hay House, 2016), p. 66.

2   Sharon Blackie, *If Women Rose Rooted: The Journey to Authenticity and Belonging* (Tewkesbury, U.K.: September Publishing, 2016), p. 13.

3   Susan Griffin. *Woman and Nature: The Roaring Inside Her* (San Francisco, CA.: Sierra Club Books, 1978), p. 34.

4   Serinity Young. *Women Who Fly: Goddesses, Witches, Mystics, and Other Airborne Females* (London, U.K.: Oxford University Press, 2018), pp. 3–4.

5   Joan Halifax. *Standing at the Edge: Finding Freedom Where Fear and Courage Meet* (New York: Flatiron Books, 2018), p. 4. According to Halifax, Edge States include altruism, empathy, integrity, respect, and engagement.

6   Lama Tsultrim Allione. *Wisdom Rising: Journey into the Mandala of the Empowered Feminine* (New York: Enliven Books, 2018), p. 108.

7   Christiane Northrup. *Women's Bodies, Women's Wisdom: Creating Physical and Emotional Health and Healing, Revised and Updated Edition* (New York: Bantam, 2006), p. 54.

8   Blackie, p. 33.

9   *The Cambridge Edition of the Works of D. H. Lawrence: Lady Chatterley's Lover and A Propos of 'Lady Chatterly's Lover' and Other Essays,* edited by Michael Squires (London, U.K.: Cambridge University Press, 2002), p. 323.

10   Ben Falk. *The Resilient Farm and Homestead: An Innovative Permaculture and Whole Systems Design Approach* (White River Junction, VT.: Chelsea Green Publishing, 2013), p. 103.

11   Sandra Ingerman and Hank Wesselman. *Awakening to the Spirit World: The Shamanic Path of Direct Revelation* (Boulder, CO.: Sounds True, 2010), p. 56.

12   Mary Reynolds Thompson. *Reclaiming the Wild Soul: How Earth's Landscapes Restore Us to Wholeness* (Ashland, OR.: White Cloud Press, 2014), p. 23.

13   Ursula Le Guin. *Buffalo Gals and Other Animal Presences* (New York: Plume/Penguin, 1987), p. 11.

14 Joan Didion. *Slouching Toward Bethlehem: Essays* (New York: Farrar, Straus and Giroux, 1961), p. 139.

15 Clarissa Pinkola Estés, *Women Who Run with the Wolves: Myths and Stories of the Wild Woman Archetype* (New York: Ballantine Books, 1992), p. 298.

16 Elizabeth Gilbert. *Big Magic: Creative Living Behind Fear* (New York: Riverhead Books, 2015), p. 13.

17 Julia Cameron. *The Artist's Way: A Spiritual Path to Higher Creativity, Twenty-Fifth Anniversary Edition* (New York: TarcherPerigee, 2016), p. 3.

18 Sharon Blackie. *If Women Rose Rooted: The Journey to Authenticity and Belonging* (Tewkesbury, U.K.: September Publishing, 2016), p. 371.

Chapter 4: Voice of the Body

1 Meggan Watterson. *Reveal: A Sacred Manual for Getting Spiritually Naked* (Carlsbad, CA.: Hay House, 2013), p. 43.

2 Susan Moon. "Body as Self," from *Being Bodies: Buddhist Women on the Paradox of Embodiment,* edited by Lenore Friedman and Susan Moon (Boston, MA.: Shambhala Publications, 1997), p. 228.

3 Zenju Earthlyn Manuel, *The Way of Tenderness: Awakening Through Race, Sexuality, and Gender* (Somerville, MA.: Wisdom Publications, 2015), p. 123.

4 Watterson.

5 Jan Chozen Bays. "Embodiment," from *Being Bodies: Buddhist Women on the Paradox of Embodiment,* edited by Lenore Friedman and Susan Moon (Boston, MA.: Shambhala, 1997), p. 172.

6 Susan Griffin, *Woman and Nature: The Roaring Inside Her* (San Francisco, CA.: Sierra Club Books, 1978), p. 303.

7 Maya Angelou. *Rainbow in the Cloud: The Wisdom and Spirit of Maya Angelou* (New York: Random House, 2014), p. 5.

8   Cynthia Orlando. "What's So Special about Oregon White Oaks?" *Forests for Oregon* (spring 2007), https://www.oregon.gov/ODF/Documents/ForestBenefits/OregonWhiteOak.pdf.

9   Sonya Renee Taylor, *The Body Is Not an Apology: The Power of Radical Self-Love* (Oakland, CA.: Berrett-Koehler Publishers, 2018), p. 3.

10 Tonya Reiman. *The Power of Body Language: How to Succeed in Every Business and Social Encounter* (New York: Simon & Schuster, 2007), pp. 37–9.

11 Reiman, p. 98.

12 Charles Duhigg. *The Power of Habit: What We Do What We Do in Life and Business* (New York: Random House, 2014), p. xvi.

13 LiYana Silver. *Feminine Genius: The Provocative Path to Waking Up and Turning on the Wisdom of Being a Woman* (Louisville, CO.: Sounds True, 2017), p. 149.

14 Golden Elixir Press website (accessed July 10, 2019) http://www.goldenelixir.com/taoism/texts_laozi_zhongjing.html. Note: This source references *Laozi zhongjing* (Central Scripture of Laozi), sec. 5. Translation published in Fabrizio Pregadio, "Early Daoist Meditation and the Origins of Inner Alchemy," in Benjamin Penny, editor, *Daoism in History: Essays in Honour of Liu Ts'un-yan,* (London, U.K.: Routledge, 2006), p. 122.

15 Daniele Martarelli, Mario Cocchioni, Stefania Scuri, and Pierluigi Pompei. "Diaphragmatic Breathing Reduces Exercise-Induced Oxidative Stress," *Evidence-Based Complementary and Alternative Medicine,* vol. 2011, article ID 932430 (Published online February 10, 2011), doi:10.1093/ecam/nep169.

16 "The Sokshing, a Sacred 'Spine'!" Dhagpo Centre Buddhiste (accessed June 21, 2019), https://stoupa.dhagpo.org/en/the-sokshing-a-sacred-spine.

17 Donna Eden with David Feinstein. *Energy Medicine: Balancing Your Body's Energies for Optimal Health, Joy, and Vitality* (New York: Penguin Group, 2008), p. 171.

[18] Jack Kornfield. *A Path with Heart: A Guide Through the Perils and Promises of Spiritual Life* (New York: Bantam Books, 1993), p. 12.

[19] HeartMath Institute. *Science of the Heart: Exploring the Role of the Heart in Human Performance,* https://www.heartmath.org/research/science-of-the-heart.

[20] Ibid.

[21] Eva Pierrakos. *The Pathwork of Self-Transformation* (New York: Bantam Books, 1990), p. xvi.

[22] Subhuti Dharmananda. *Towards a Spirit at Peace: Understanding the Treatment of Shen Disorders with Chinese Medicine* (Portland, OR.: Institute for Traditional Medicine and Preventive Health Care, 2005), https://www.itmonline.org/shen.

[23] Diane Ackerman. *The Moon by Whale Light and Other Adventures Among Bats, Penguins, Crocodilians, and Whales* (New York: Random House, 1991), p. 177.

[24] Desmond Morris. *The Human Animal: A Personal View of the Human Species* (New York: Crown, 1994), p. 130.

[25] Jacob Israel Liberman. *Luminous Life: How the Science of Light Unlocks the Art of Living* (Novato, CA.: New World Library, 2018), p. 25.

[26] Liberman, pp. 25–6.

[27] Olivia Kang and Thalia Wheatley. "Pupil Dilation Patterns Spontaneously Synchronize across Individuals during Shared Attention," *Journal of Experimental Psychology: General,* vol. 146, no. 4 (2017), pp. 569–76.

[28] Leil Lowndes. *How to Instantly Connect with Anyone: 96 All-New Little Tricks for Big Success in Relationships,* (New York: McGraw-Hill, 2009), pp. 3–5.

Chapter 5: Sacred Initiations

[1] L.R. Knost, as cited in Mary Bea Sullivan. *Living the Way of Love: A 40-Day Devotional* (New York: Church Publishing, 2019), p. 90.

2   Rebecca Solnit. *The Faraway Nearby* (New York: Penguin Books, 2013), pp. 3–4.

3   Rick Hanson. *Hardwiring Happiness: The New Brain Science of Contentment, Calm and Confidence* (New York: Harmony, 2016), pp. 17–31.

4   Emily Hancock. "The Girl Within: Touchstone for Women's Identity," from *To Be a Woman: The Birth of the Conscious Feminine,* edited by Connie Zweig (New York: G.P. Putnam, New York, 1990), pp. 56–7.

5   Ibid., p. 62.

6   "Rod of Asclepius," Wikipedia.com (accessed September 30, 2019).

7   Jeanette LeBlanc. "You Are Not Alone," personal blog (accessed September 30, 2019), https://www.jeanetteleblanc.com/you-are-not-alone.

8   Pema Chödrön. *When Things Fall Apart: Heart Advice for Difficult Times* (Boston: Shambhala Publications, 2000), p. 7.

9   "Failure," Merriam-Webster.com (accessed June 22, 2019).

10 "The Perils of Perfectionism," *Harvard Mental Health Newsletter* (November 2007), www.health.harvard.edu/newsletter_article/The_perils_of_perfectionism.

11 Richard R. Powell. *Wabi Sabi Simple: Create Beauty. Value Imperfection. Live Deeply* (Avon, MA.: Adams Media, 2004), p. 6.

12 Robyn Griggs Lawrence, *The Wabi-Sabi House: The Japanese Art of Imperfect Beauty* (New York: Clarkson Potter Publishers, 2004), p. 17.

13 Ibid.

14 Common Dreams Staff. "German Study: Alarming Levels of Dangerous Plastics in Children's Bodies," CommonDreams.org (September 14, 2019).

15 Katty Kay and Clare Shipman. *The Confidence Code: The Science and Art of Self-Assurance-What Women Should Know* (New York: Harper Collins, 2014), p. 40.

[16] Nansook Park. "The Role of Subjective Well-being in Positive Youth Development," *Annals of the American Academy of Political and Social Science,* vol. 591, no. 1 (2004), pp. 25–39.

[17] Carol Dweck, as cited by James Morehead. "Stanford University's Carol Dweck on the Growth Mindset and Education," OneDublin.org (June 19, 2012).

[18] Ibid.

[19] Rachel Simmons. *Enough as She Is: How to Help Girls Move Beyond Impossible Standards of Success to Live Healthy, Happy, and Fulfilling Lives* (New York: HarperCollins, 2018), p. 88.

[20] Virginia Woolf, as cited in Serinity Young. *Women Who Fly: Goddesses, Witches, Mystics, and Other Airborne Females* (New York: Oxford University Press, 2018), p. 103.

[21] "Five Things That Will Improve Your Life in 2013," CarolineMiller.com (accessed June 22, 2019).

[22] Hunter Drohojowska-Philp. *Full Bloom: The Art and Life of Georgia O'Keeffe* (New York: W.W. Norton, 2004), p. 213.

Chapter 6: Anoint Yourself

[1] Sharon Salzberg. *Real Love: The Art of Mindful Connection* (New York: Flatiron Books, 2017). p. 4.

[2] Tsultrim Allione. *Wisdom Rising: Journey into the Mandala of the Empowered Feminine* (New York: Enliven Books, 2018), p.15.

[3] Danielle LaPorte. *The White Hot Truth* (Vancouver, B.C, Canada: Virtuonica, 2017), p. 65.

[4] Frans de Waal. *The Age of Empathy: Nature's Lessons for a Kinder Society* (New York: Harmony Books, 2018), p. 9.

[5] Ibid., p. 10-11.

[6] Ibid., p. 208.

[7] Valarie Kaur. "Three Lessons of Revolutionary Love in a Time of Rage," TED.com (accessed November 21, 2019).

8   Ibid.

9   Aluna Joy Yaxkin. "In Lak'ech Ala K'in - the Living Code of the Heart," Aluna Joy (November 2007), https://www.alunajoy.com/2007nov.html.

10 Valarie Kaur website (accessed July 10, 2019), http://valariekaur.com.

11 Ed Yong. "How Chimpanzees Deal with Death and Dying," NationalGeographic.com (April 26, 2010).

12 Thom van Dooren. "Mourning Crows: Grief and Extinction in a Shared World," *Routledge Handbook of Human-Animal Studies,* edited by Garry Marvin and Susan McHugh (New York: Routledge, 2014).

13 Laura Parker. "Rare Footage: Wild Elephants 'Mourn' Their Dead," NationalGeographic.com (August 31, 2016).

14 Jenny Gathright. "After 17 Days and 1,000 miles, a Mother Orca's 'Tour of Grief' Is Over," NPR.org (August 12, 2018).

15 Lynda Mapes. "Orca Tahlequah is a Mother Again," SeattleTimes.com (September 5, 2020).

16 Chögyam Trungpa Rinpoche, as cited by Ram Dass. *Polishing the Mirror: How to Live from our Spiritual Heart* (Boulder, CO.: Sounds True, 2013), p. 74.

17 Suzanne W. Simard. "Mycorrhizal Networks Facilitate Tree Communication, Learning, and Memory," in *Memory and Learning in Plants,* edited by Frantisek Baluska, Monica Gagliano, and Guenther Witzany (New York: Springer, International Publishing, 2018), pp. 191–213.

18 Kamala Masters. "The Preciousness of Our Human Life," Vipassana Metta on Maui (accessed June 21, 2019), http://vipassanametta.org/wp/wp-content/uploads/2012/01/The-Preciousness-of-Our-Human-Life.pdf.

19 Natalie Goldberg. *Writing Down the Bones: Freeing the Writer Within* (Boulder, CO.: Shambhala Publications, 1986), p. 8.

Chapter 7: Waters of Restorations

[1] Debbie Ford. *Courage: Overcoming Fear and Igniting Self-Confidence* (New York; HarperCollins Publishers, 2012), pp. 52, 54.

[2] Ed Yong. "Octopus Cares for Her Eggs for 53 Months, Then Dies," NationalGeographic.com (July 30, 2014).

[3] C.G. Jung. *Spirit in Man, Art, and Literature,* edited and translated by Gerhard Adler and R.F.C. Hull (Princeton, N.J.: Princeton University Press, 1966), p. 4.

[4] Marianne Williamson. *A Woman's Worth* (New York: Ballantine Books, 1993), p. 53.

[5] Clarissa Pinkola Estés. *Women Who Run with the Wolves: Myths and Stories of the Wild Woman Archetype* (New York: Ballantine Books, 1992), p. 256.

[6] Lori Eve Dechar. *Five Spirits: Alchemical Acupuncture for Psychological and Spiritual Healing* (Brooklyn, N.Y.: Lantern Books, 2006), pp. 275–6.

[7] "Dadirri," Yarra Healing (accessed June 21, 2019), http://www.yarrahealing.catholic.edu.au/celebrations/index.cfm?loadref=58.

[8] "Astonish," Etymology Online, https://www.etymonline.com/word/astonish.

[9] "From the Vault: Tony Robbins and Deepak Chopra," Tony Robbins (accessed July 10, 2019), https://www.tonyrobbins.com/podcasts/vault-tony-robbins-deepak-chopra.

Deep Bows

[1] Katagiri Roshi, as cited by Natalie Goldberg. *Writing Down the Bones: Freeing the Writer Within* (Boulder, CO.: Shambhala Publications, 1986), p. 16.

RESOURCES

Thank you for sharing these pages with me. It is my hope that you continue to live a reclamation of self-trust through the guidance of the living world. Here, everything happens in its natural unfolding. Here, all of you belongs.

It would be an honor for us to continue working together in the spirit of change and renewal. You can visit KendraWard.com to learn more about:

Online Teachings
Cocreative courses that explore our intrapsychic drive to know the wilderness of our souls.

Join My Pack
Explore my free offerings and sign-up for my monthly missives.

Stay in Touch
Facebook: kendraward.rewild
Instagram: @kendra.a.ward

ABOUT THE AUTHOR

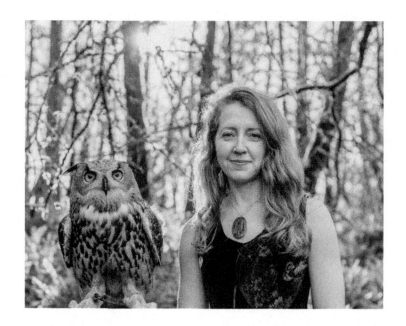

Kendra Ward, L.Ac., MAOM, is a traditional Chinese medicine practitioner and herbalist. From 2003 to 2020, she co-owned the Whole Family Wellness Center in Portland, Oregon, immersing herself in a busy private practice with over 25,000 patient visits.

Kendra's primary teachers are not the long-dead figures of history or dogma, but the land where she lives, her lifelong meditation and spiritual practices, and the complex, honest, radiant human beings she has been fortunate to hold space for in her healing practice.

Kendra's writing has an ecospiritual, Earth-honoring focus and has been featured in *Yes!*, *Nature Evolutionaries*, *Rebelle Society*, *Elephant Journal*, and elsewhere. *Throwing Thunder* is her first book.

Kendra now lives with her family in western Vermont, which is the unceded territory of the Abenaki peoples. When she is not in the clinic or writing, you can find her conversing with the many barred owls in the forests near her home.

Made in the USA
Las Vegas, NV
12 August 2022

53154237R10134